KU-014-785

Economic Evaluation of Health Care in Developing Countries

THEORY AND APPLICATIONS

Guy Carrin

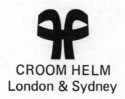

CROOM HELM
London & Sydney

ST. MARTIN'S PRESS
New York

© 1984 Guy Carrin
Croom Helm Ltd, Provident House, Burrell Row,
Beckenham, Kent BR3 1AT

Croom Helm Australia Pty Ltd, GPO Box 5097,
Sydney, NSW 2001, Australia

British Library Cataloguing in Publication Data

Carrin, Guy
    Economic evaluation of health care in developing
    countries.
    1. Developing countries — Medical care
    2. Developing countries — Medical economics
    I. Title
    338.4'73621'091724   RA410.5

    ISBN 0-7099-0786-9

All rights reserved. For information, write:
St. Martin's Press, Inc., 175 Fifth Avenue, New York, NY 10010
First published in the United States of America in 1984

Library of Congress Cataloging in Publication Data

Carrin, Guy.
    Economic evaluation of health care in developing
countries

    Includes index.
     1. Medical care — Developing countries — Evaluation.
2. Medical economics — Developing countries. I. Title.
[DNLM: 1. Health services — Economics. 2. Developing
countries. 3. Health. WA 395 C318e]
RA399.D44C37   1984   362.1'042   83-23068
ISBN 0-312-23231-4 (St. Martin's Press)

Printed and bound in Great Britain

CONTENTS

FOREWORD

The "genuine" tropical doctor is a Jack of all trades. This includes a role as health administrator and health promotor. These responsibilities impose a direct involvement or a close contact with the budgetary planning of health services. For that purpose he needs a comprehensive view of health determinants, and of a constructive analytical approach to cost-benefit, cost-effectiveness and similar economic ingredients. His main problem is not an awareness of the financial implications of health care, but an ability to discuss in a common understandable language with the economic counsellors of the decision-makers. Preaching to deaf ears leaves both sides in a frustrated mood.

The "World Health Organization", which is the efficient motor for the development of health planning, became from the very beginning of its activities aware of the need for some sort of medico-economic understanding and the difficulties in getting it to work.

As far as the "Country Health Programming" is concerned, 23 countries had started such a program when the Director General reported to the General Assembly in 1978. Since then many more countries showed interest.

Concerning specific disease-, sanitation-oriented action programs neither U.N. or other international agencies, nor prospective contributors accept any longer to participate in health programs on mere humanitarian motives. They require a reasonable evidence of a positive relation between health improvement and economic growth. This aspect received much attention from WHO but, except for a

few attempts of promoting an understanding between
public health experts and health-conscious economists
or for the use of economists as consultants, no for-
mal medico-economic unit has been established.

The Special Programme for Research and Training
in Tropical Diseases (TDR) decided to include a socio-economic unit, which was the last to come about,
but is by now very active.

In the meantime, health economists have forced
themselves upon the medical profession of the indus-
trialized world. However problems related to the
rapid generalization of expensive new, advanced
technologies and sophisticated treatments are quite
different from those which could help in the long
battle for a brighter future for health in less developed countries (LDC's).

The "Francqui Foundation", Brussels (Belgium),
aware of this discrepancy, decided to fund generous-
ly a survey on the specific medico-economic
problems characteristic of the less developed countries. On the basis of the collected data, together
with much study, discussions, thinking and testing
out on real situations, Guy Carrin wrote this excellent manual.

The economist had to familiarize himself with
health concepts and indicators, medical terminology
and way of thinking. He is now inviting the medical
profession and overseas health administrators to
come at grips with an economic jargon and economically sound approaches of the health problems in
LDC's.

An interested reader of this practice oriented
and clear exposition of the basic health problem
will get convinced of his capacity to absorb the
health development approach as seen by an economist.
A logical build-up of well-adapted knowledge leads
to health-planning, providing meanwhile with a new
terminology and a conviction that a growth build up
on a "basic needs" approach is an efficient way of
attacking poor health in LDC's.

Health-planning is presented in a stepwise
manner along different stages: data collection,
their analysis, identification of critical areas
and constraints, preparation of and decision on the
proposed program, its integration in the country's

health structures. Targets are to be set as much as possible in accordance with the felt needs and preferences of the population.

The choice of the evaluation methods present ed will as a matter of course be influenced by the availability of information, the needs and by the preferences of those concerned: cost-benefit, cost-effectiveness, multiattribute problem analysis, linear programming, regression analysis, econometric modeling.

The handbook, completed by appendices, contains carefully selected realistic case studies and a wealth of information generally dispersed over many publications. They will turn out to be a fertile ground for reflexion, setting up of policy alternatives, design of scenario's illustrating the relations between health and economics.

The duty of the health administrators and policy-makers being the most efficient use of scarce resources, this manual will support them strongly in performing their difficult, but exalting task.

Prof.em.Dr.P.G.JANSSENS
Honorary-director of the
Institute for Tropical
Medicine "Prince Leopold"-
Antwerp

PREFACE

This book is the result of a research project on the economic evaluation of health interventions in developing countries. The book first presents an assessment of the basic health problems in developing countries in Part I. The first chapter studies the determinants of poor health while the second chapter discusses the linkages between health and economic development. It is strongly recommended to read these chapters before continuing with the study of Part II on methods for economic evaluation in health care. The main reason is that economic evaluation methods can only be applied fruitfully in developing countries if one understands the causes of poor health and the intertwinement between health and the economy. In chapters three to eight, a study is made of cost-benefit analysis, cost-effectiveness analysis, multiattribute problem analysis, linear programming, regression analysis and policy evaluation, respectively. The last chapter of Part II discusses health planning in developing countries as advocated by the WHO.

The various topics in this book are presented basically at the undergraduate level. Part I does not require special knowledge of economics, mathematics or statistics. Part II presumes some familiarity with basic economic concepts, calculus and matrix algebra, however. Throughout the book we want to emphasize the applicability of the evaluation methods. That is why the reader will encounter many examples and case-studies while studying the material.

The book is destined for two kinds of readers: first, for public health administrators and doctors with a responsibility and/or interest in evaluation

Preface

of health care in the third world, and, secondly,
for students of economics, medicine and public
health who desire to acquire knowledge about the
essentials of economic evaluation of health interventions.

The research on this book was supervised by
Professors P.G.Janssens and W.Nonneman of the Institute of Tropical Medecine (Antwerp, Belgium) and
the University of Antwerp (UFSIA), respectively.
They always encouraged me during the effort of writing this book,by supplying information, by discussing with me various issues in the field of health
economics or by commenting on previous drafts of the
book. I sincerely thank them for their help. I am
also grateful to Professor J.Vuylsteke for the many
discussions we had; because of his wide field experience in developing countries, each discussion
proved to be a new source of information and inspi-
ration. I am also very much indebted to I.Decancq-
Van Gaelen and H. De Craen for transmitting useful
information to me. W. Kennes,J. Van Dael, Dr. R.
Renard, Professor M. Tharakan and two anonymous ref-
erees are thanked sincerely for reading and commenting upon earlier versions of a number of chapters.

The members of the administative staff of the
Studiecentrum voor Economisch en Sociaal Onderzoek,
A. Bunneghem, L. Gysels and K. Van den broeck joined
cheerfully and very competently in the production
of this book. A. Bunneghem drew the graphs and was
very helpful in proofreading and making the index.
L. Gysels typed several chapters of earlier versions
of the book. K. Van den broeck undertook the major
and tedious task of typing several versions of the
whole manuscript. She was also responsible for the
lay-out of the book. I thank all of them most sincerely for their proficient collaboration. I also
express my gratitude to my home institution, the
University of Antwerp (UFSIA) for giving me a grant
towards the publication of this book. Last but not
least, I remain indebted to my wife Rita and my
children Maarten, Jeroen and Marijs for their support; their love made the writing of this book all
the more worthwhile.

Guy CARRIN
SESO

TABLES AND FIGURES

Tables

Figures

PART I

AN ASSESSMENT OF THE CAUSES OF POOR HEALTH

IN DEVELOPING COUNTRIES

Chapter One

DETERMINANTS OF HEALTH

1.1. INTRODUCTION

1.1.1. THE UNEQUAL DISTRIBUTION OF HEALTH IN THE WORLD

Without doubt good health is a basic goal common to
all of mankind. Yet as can be seen from Table 1.1,
health is distributed rather unequally. In this
table the three variables measuring health status
are life expectancy at birth in years (LIFE), the
infant mortality rate of children aged 0 to 1 (IM)
and the child death rate of children 1 to 5 (CD).

One notices that the developing world, including the oil exporters, is worse off than the developed world in terms of life expectancy. A comparison of the data on infant and child mortality rein-
forces the finding that the developing world is
characterized by an inferior health status. The
major reason is evidently that scarcity of resources represents a basic and severe constraint on
many less developed countries (LDC), whence the resources that are allocated to health are frequently
insufficient. One has to understand that, apart
from achieving better health conditions, developing
countries have a whole set of other objectives to
meet. For instance, objectives such as industrial
and agricultural growth will frequently demand resources at the expense of an improvement in health
conditions. Economic growth will now gradually alleviate the constraint on resources, so that one
can expect that over time more resources will be
spent on health care. *A fortiori*, it is then also
to be expected that economic growth will contribute
indirectly to a better health status. In order to
verify the latter, admittedly in a crude way, we
will inspect by means of a scatter diagram the re-

lation between life expectancy and gross national product per capita (GNP). In drawing Figure 1.1 we have made use of World Bank data for 100 LDC[1].

Figure 1.1 clearly shows that increases in life expectancy accompany increases in GNP. Two important remarks are in order here. *First,* economic progress cannot buy continuous improvement in life expectancy. Around the age of 70 the marginal effect of GNP becomes rather small. Countries with a high life expectancy can then only hope that economic progress will contribute to lower morbidity levels. *Secondly,* some countries with rather high GNP levels such as Saudi Arabia and Libya have a low life expectancy. The opposite is also true, namely that some poor countries such as Sri Lanka and China have a high life expectancy. The latter obviously leads to a realization that economic progress, as measured by GNP, is not to be seen as the major direct determinant of health. In fact we have to realize that GNP hides a number of true health determinants. The study of these health determinants forms the core of this chapter.

Table 1.1. A comparison of health status data between less developed and developed countries, in 1980

Type of economy	GNP (in US $)	LIFE (in years)	IM (‰)	CD (‰)
Low-income developing economies	260	57	94	12
China and India	270	59	84	10
Other low-income	230	48	130	22
Middle-income developing economies	1,400	60	80	11
Oil exporters	1,160	56	94	14
Oil importers	1,580	63	69	9
High-income oil exporters (Libya,Saudi Arabia,Kuwait, United Arab Emirates)	12,630	57	99	14
Industrial Market Economies	10,320	74	11	1
Nonmarket Industriel Economies	4,640	71	25	1

Source: World Bank (1982), Statistical Appendix.

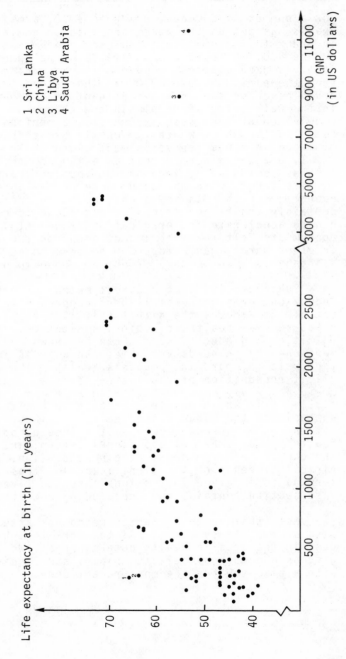

Figure 1.1. Relationship between life expectancy at birth (in years) and GNP (in US dollars) in 1980

1 Sri Lanka
2 China
3 Libya
4 Saudi Arabia

Determinants of health

1.1.2. HEALTH IMPROVEMENT: THE BASIC NEEDS VIEW

For a number of decades, prior to 1970, a major emphasis was put on the need for rapid economic growth in order to improve the social and economic situation in the LDC. Since the early 1970s, development objectives have changed, however. A major conclusion from the period before 1970 was that economic growth could never be the only determinant of improvement in the well-being of people in the LDC. For fast growing countries, such as Brazil[2], a serious dispute started about whether economic growth had diminished absolute impoverishment among the poor. Still, one could notice that in a few countries, such as South Korea, income distribution improved simultaneously with the occurrence of a vigorous economic growth. In any event, although one could certainly prove theoretically that economic growth had to accelerate the eradication of poverty, many economists felt that its impact occurred too slowly. In other words, many stopped to believe in an instantaneous trickle-down effect of economic growth.

Subsequently, a more direct method of poverty reduction, namely the basic needs approach was advocated: its aim was the direct fulfillment of basic needs such as health, clothing, sanitation, shelter, nutrition and education. It can be shown that the mentioned basic needs variables can play an important role in improving people's health. The explicit recognition of the latter leads then to a *basic needs approach to health improvement*. Essentially it is an integrated approach to health care emphasizing that inadequate health services[3] are not the only cause of poor health. Indeed, poor health has a number of additional determinants; those will be discussed in the next section. Empirical evidence on the significance of these determinants is given in sections three to five. The last section contains some concluding remarks.

Note that in this chapter we do not attempt to give a complete survey of all the work that has been done in the area of health determinants. We will discuss a number of selected papers and findings, with a bias towards the most recent ones.

1.2. MAJOR DETERMINANTS OF POOR HEALTH[4]

1.2.1. POPULATION GROWTH

In most LDC fertility rates are fairly high and contribute to a number of health problems on the family level. High fertility among poor households is the main cause of crowded housing. In turn the latter gives rise to a high disease rate and increased problems of insanitation. Fertility rates and mortality as well as morbidity rates are therefore correlated. Given the fact that children are less immune to disease than adults, morbidity and mortality rates among children are especially high. Note that high child mortality will usually reinforce the fertility rate. Indeed, high child mortality incites low income parents to choose a high fertility rate, in order to ensure that they will be supported by a sufficient number of children during their old age.

High fertility can also have a large impact on the economy in general. In many countries, agriculture is not well developed so that fertility will have a negative effect on food availability per capita. Population pressure may also slow down agricultural development when it leads to overcropping and soil degradation[5]. In addition high birth rates will make government planning of various social services more difficult. The higher the birth rate, the higher the cost of medical services, since more medical personnel have to be trained eventually. It will also be more difficult to provide adequate clean water supply, garbage disposal and adequate housing for the entire population if population pressure is high.

It is clear, given the above, that population planning is one of the ingredients of a health care programme of a developing country. The coverage of population planning should of course be as wide as possible. Attention should be paid therefore to coverage of rural areas. This implies that communities need to be involved, for instance, in family planning education and in the distribution of contraceptives[6].

1.2.2. MALNUTRITION[7]

Malnutrition is one of the principal causes of pre-

mature death in developing countries. Much of the
literature on malnutrition focuses on the relationship between nutrition and the health of children,
since the latter constitute an especially vulnerable group.

Winikoff and Brown (1980) discuss a number of
principal determinants of health of children in developing countries. *First,* birth weight, that is
an important predictor of childhood health, is correlated positively with a number of measures of maternal nutrition; among these variables we include
measures of long-standing nutritional status (maternal height and prepregnant weight) and maternal
nutrition during pregnancy (represented by maternal
weight gain during gestation). Improving maternal
nutrition is therefore likely to decrease infant
mortality. *Secondly,* childhood nutritional status
(measured by weight-for-age or weight gain over time)
is correlated negatively with the mortality rate of
children. Here two particular nutritional risks are
distinguished. The first risk is that of inadequate
infant feeding. More particularly, if babies do not
receive breast-feeding, which is the appropriate
method of nutrition:
(i) they loose the protective anti-infective prop-
erties of mothers' milk;
(ii) they run the risk of being fed inadequate and/
or contaminated food.
The second nutritional risk is at the age of weaning. Marginally nourished mothers can breast-feed
their children during the first months of a child's
life without causing child malnutrition. To rely on
breast-feeding along after a period of six months
is insufficient to maintain the child's health,
however. Supplemental foods are therefore necessary.
In poor areas, the latter are often unavailable,
causing the period of weaning to be dangerous for
the child's nutritional status. *Thirdly,* the mother's parity and age may influence infant mortality,
namely children of a higher birth order are also
likely to have a greater mortality risk. Also the
sex of the child is often a contributing factor to
the child's mortality risk: countries or areas where
parents have a preference for sons usually show a
lower nutritional and health status for female children[8].

1.2.3. SANITARY CONDITIONS AND INADEQUATE SHELTER

Many infectious diseases in LDC such as typhoid, dysentery and cholera are caused by unsafe drinking water and contaminated food. Water and food get contaminated quite easily when human or animal excreta are not adequately disposed of. The diseases that are caused by the poor bacteriological quality of the water are called *water-borne diseases*[9].

The lack of personal hygiene and poor sanitation is a particular cause of acute enteric and parasitic diseases,trachoma, conjunctivitis and various skin infections. For these diseases, the insufficient water volume is assumed to be more important than the bacteriological quality of water. These diseases are called *water-washed diseases*[10]. It is evident, however, that better hygienic practices need to accompany a better supply of clean water in order to depress the disease rate.

Some diseases are caused by organisms that live in soil that is contaminated by feaces. For instance, in the events of a poor sanitary environment in which many people are bare-footed, the larvae of hookworms can enter the body through the skin of the feet and subsequently infect the human body. Such diseases are called *fecal disposal diseases*. Inadequate shelter is also a factor determining frequently the incidence of *airborne diseases* such as tuberculosis; indeed, overcrowding stimulates the transmission of such diseases. Programs for better housing are therefore bound to improve health among the poor population.

1.2.4. EDUCATION

Lack of education or information about the benefits of adequate nutrition, personal hygiene, clean water supply and waste disposal may seriously hamper the health status of individuals. In the case of nutrition of infants, for instance, information should be given about the benefits of breast-feeding[11]: it improves children's health because the milk of the mother is of high nutritional value and because it improves children's resistance to diseases. Another benefit of breast-feeding is that lactational amenorrhea is a rather effective method of birth control. Concerning water supply and waste disposal, instruction about the proper use of unpolluted water and toilet facilities and about correct hygienic habits is an essential ingredient of health intervention policies.

1.2.5. DISEASE CONTROL

As already said above, parasitic and other infectious diseases[12] can be decreased if better sanitation facilities and more adequate clean water supply become available. Better nutrition can also be a contributory factor of a declining infectious disease rate.

Immunizations are effective in combatting childhood diseases such as measles, polio, tetanus, diphteria and pertussis. In the case of *vector-borne* tropical diseases[13] such as malaria, sleeping sickness (trypanosomiasis), schistosomiasis and riverblindness (onchocerciasis), control of the vector is an obvious method to depress the tropical disease rate. There are also efficient drugs against many tropical diseases.

Note that the diseases that are transmitted by insects that breed in water or bite near it (malaria, riverblindness, sleeping sickness, yellow fever, filariasis, etc.), are also called *water-vectored diseases*[14]. The diseases that are transmitted by a vector which spends part of its life cycle in water (e.g. schistosomiasis) are called *water-based diseases*[15].

1.2.6. HEALTH SERVICES

Most LDC lack sufficient availability of medical personnel and medical infrastructure, such as general hospitals and rural clinics. Two remarks are to be made. *First,* medical personnel should not be seen as restricted to physicians and nurses. It also includes midwives, auxiliary nurses and community health workers. In fact the latter can be as effective as physicians in a number of cases. It should also be emphasized here that medical personnel ought to receive a training which is geared to specific needs in developing countries. For instance, a one sided curative orientation in medical training signifies in most instances a waste of resources. *Secondly,* the mere availability of techniques of modern medicine (such as drugs) does not guarantee a positive long-term effect on the health of the population: if the environment in which people live remains unhealthy, drugs can bring at best only temporary relief from diseases.

It is now widely recognized that a main emphasis has to be put on preventive services, easy access to health care and improvements in the other determinants of health discussed above. Organizations such as WHO, UNICEF and the World Bank agree upon the necessity of *primary health care*. The latter term refers to health care that 'adresses the main health problems in the community, providing promotive, preventive, curative and rehabilitative services accordingly' and it 'includes at least: education concerning prevailing health problems and the methods of preventing and controlling them; promotion of food supply and proper nutrition; and adequate supply of safe water and basic sanitation; maternal and child health care, including diseases; prevention and control of locally endemic diseases; appropriate treatment of common diseases and injuries; and provision of essential drugs'[16].

1.3. EMPIRICAL EVIDENCE FROM MICRO-STUDIES ON THE EFFECT OF HEALTH DETERMINANTS[17]

1.3.1. DEMOGRAPHIC FACTOR

Lowering the population growth in the LDC would alleviate the health problems in those areas. A major consequence would be that more food would become available per person, so that the nutritional status would be enhanced and the susceptibility to diseases decreased. Among the studies that show the necessity of fertility decline, we first cite Morley *et al.* (1968) and Gopalan and Rao (1969). They show that there exists a negative correlation between a large family size and close spacing of births on the one hand and food availability and care to children on the other hand. These studies were done in Nigeria and India respectively. In Wray (1971), similar evidence for Thailand is reported. Kunstadter (1978) also reports on evidence that higher birth order children have a higher mortality risk; a number of calculations reveal that mothers of very high parity (up to 20 children) have a high probability that only 10 children will survive. This mortality risk does not seem to stop with infancy; children of high parity mothers remain

11

at a greater risk throughout childhood. Kunstadter, found that mortality of children whose mother's parity is above the mean for their age is nearly twice as high as the mortality of those children whose mothers are below mean parity[18].

Chowdhury (1974) has found that, in rural Bangladesh, there is a negative relationship between birth-spacing and post-neonatal mortality rates. Namely, 'if the previous infant was alive, and the next birth came in less that 26 months, the post-neonatal mortality rate for the next birth was 95 per cent higher than if the next birth was delayed beyond 26 months'[19]. Chowdhury attributes this differential to the competition for food by the succeeding child. In addition Omran and Standley (1976) found that children born in Asia and the Near East within a year after their previous sibling have a mortality risk that is 2 to 4 times as high as that of children that are born 3 years or more after a previous birth. Similar findings are reported by Mata (1978) for Guatemala: the probability of survival of children born between 9 to 17 months after a previous birth is low both during the first 4 weeks and the first 6 months of life, respectively. There is also evidence communicated by Puffer and Serrano (1973) about childhood mortality in Recife, Brazil: 14 per cent of first and second born children deceased whereas 51 per cent of fifth and later-born children died[20].

1.3.2. NUTRITION[21]

Table 1.2 suggests that in some Latin American areas nutritional deficiency is a significant *direct cause of death*; see especially the figures for Columbia and El Salvador. Notice that together with an associated cause (measles, diarrhea, respiratory cause etc.), malnutrition is an important death determining factor. A study on the role of malnutrition in child mortality has been done by Sommer and Loewenstein(1975). A nutritional survey of 8292 children (aged 1 to 9) was conducted in the Matlab area (Bangladesh) at the end of 1970. The nutritional status of these children was measured by a ratio of arm circumference to height. It was concluded that 41 per cent and 9 per cent were moderately and severely malnourished, respectively. The health status of 98.8 per cent of these children was verified, 18 months later. The overall mortality rate was 2.3

per cent, but the severely malnourished children had a death rate 3.4 times higher than the
adequately nourished groups[22].

Table 1.2. Malnutrition as primary or associated
cause in deaths of children under age 5,
selected areas,1971

Area	Per cent of Deaths caused by Malnutrition		
	Primary cause	Associated cause	Primary or Associated cause
Argentina			
Chaco Province			
Resistencia	7	57	64
Rural	3	48	51
Brazil			
Recife	6	60	66
Sao Paulo	6	45	51
Colombia			
Cali	16	40	56
Medellin	11	51	62
Jamaica			
Kingston	6	32	38
Bolivia			
La Paz	4	41	45
Mexico			
Monterrey	4	48	52
Chile			
Santiago	6	39	45
El Salvador			
San Salvador	9	49	58
Rural	14	44	58

Source: Puffer and Serrano (1973, p.A183); also
presented in Sorkin (1976, pp.28-29).

Malnutrition is also a crucial element in explaining the *disease rate*. Scrimshaw *et al*. (1968)
found that the incidence of tuberculosis is much
lower among adequately nourished populations. Puffer
and Serrano (1973) observed also that in Recife
(Brazil) 74 per cent of measles deaths were associated with nutritional deficiency. If the latter increases the susceptibility to various diseases, one
says that there is a *synergistic* relationship between
infection and malnutrition[23]. Scrimshaw *et al*.
(1968) state very clearly[24] that in such a situation
'simultaneous presence of malnutrition and infection

13

results in an interaction that is more serious for the host than could be expected from the combined effect of the two working independently'.

An example of this synergistic relationship is that diarrheal diseases are followed a couple of weeks later by the increased incidence of nutrional diseases. Indeed, diarrhea makes the absorption of food more difficult, so that increased food intake is required in order to maintain a minimum nutrional status. Scrimshaw *et al.* (1968, pp.216-221) illustrate this synergistic relationship by referring to studies in Mexico, India and Brazil. An interesting study[25] is that by Wray (1977) on the effect of a nutritional program on the incidence of diarrhea among preschoolers in Cali, Columbia. In this program, each malnourished preschool child was provided with a weekly ration of one pound of dried skimmed milk. In addition, mothers were given basic education about the ways of preventing malnutrition. One result of this program was that 70 per cent of the children in the sample saw their nutritional status improved. Another result was that the diarrheal disease rate dropped significantly during the study period. Another piece of evidence is that given by Taylor *et al.* (1978) who studied the impact of nutrition supplement and medical care on children's weight in the Narangwal experimental project; note that children's weight can be considered as a health indicator. This impact was found to be positive and statistically significant[26].

The importance of *breast-feeding* for the child's health status is demonstrated by a number of studies. For instance, Yayasuriya and Soysa (1974) studied the effects of breast milk and three different milk preparations on the early growth of low-birth-weight new-borns. The death rate among those babies that were formula-fed varied from 20 to 23 per cent; the death rate among the breast-fed babies was nil. A similar study was done by Chandra (1979, p.692) in a rural Indian community on infection-related morbidity of infants. There was evidence that breast-fed infants were clearly less prone to such disorders as respiratory infection, otitis, diarrhea, dehydration and pneumonia than formula-fed infants[27].

We should also mention the possibility of a negative impact of malnutrition on body growth.

For instance, in India it was found that 90 per cent of a group of 3000 low socioeconomic children, who have a high probability of being malnourished, were below the norm of height and weight for healthy children[28]. Note that malnutrition among children also affects the brain's growth[29]. Malnutrition of pregnant and lactating women can also damage the fetus[30]. One is also likely to find a negative relationship between malnutrition and intellectual capacity[31]. However, it is agreed upon that an environment of general deprivation is the main cause of low intellectual capacity. Malnutrition is therefore only one determinant of an impaired intellectual development[32]. There is now some controversy on the reversibility of potential negative effects of malnutrition at the early stages of development of the fetus and the child. While for instance Scrimshaw (1967) and Winnick and Rosso (1969) claim that malnutrition before the age of two is irreversible, Kugelmass *et al.* (1944) found that treatment for malnutrition in the early years resulted in IQ increases from 10 to 18 per cent. Clearly, more research is needed here, but the general conclusion still seems to be that malnutrition is likely to influence the future social and economic position of malnourished children[33].

1.3.3. SANITATION AND HOUSING

The positive effect of *good sanitary conditions* on the state of health is illustrated by a number of studies. Van Zijl (1966) found that for several developing countries adequate water supply and better sanitation facilities bring down the diarrheal disease rate . Schliessman (1959) noted that privy construction in Costa Rica halved the death rate from diarrhea and enteritis between 1942 and 1954. In the Philippines, the Philippines Cholera Committee (1971) reported that better water supply and toilet facilities decreased the cholera incidence by 70 per cent. Koopman (1978) found that if schools in Cali, Columbia, would create hygienic toilet conditions, diarrhea and vomiting among schoolchildren would be reduced by 44 per cent and 34 per cent respectively.

We must emphasize that improved sanitary conditions can only have a beneficial effect if the population makes use of the improvements. In other words the social environment must be such that it

can *absorb* the improvements: people must have the
proper education and knowledge about water use and
hygiene. For instance, it must be understood by
people that they should not only use clean water
for drinking but also for preparing food. They are
also supposed to stop using polluted water for personal hygiene etc. The fact that increased water
supply and waste disposal needs to be implemented
simultaneously with other general sanitation measures is indicated by the following studies. Stanley (1977) reports that in Lesotho a rural water
supply program had no health benefits, because
people were not instructed about the beneficial use
of unpolluted water systems. The same conclusion
was reached by Rajasekaran (1977) in a study of
protected water systems of five Indian villages.
Levine *et al*. (1976) and Curlin *et al*. (1977) observed that in an area of Bangladesh, the availability of uncontaminated tubewell water did not depress
the cholera or diarrhea incidence rate. The reason
was that village residents continued to use surface
water 'for bathing, food preparation, utensil washing and water for ablution following defecation'[34].

Regarding waste disposal, the installation of
toilets may have no or even a negative effect on
health[35]. Without a minimum of sanitary education,
privies are not maintained as they should; sometimes, they are used as chicken coops or grain stor-
age facilities. It is evident that in such cases
the marginal impact on health is minimum[36].
In another study, the effects of three different
types of interventions were quantified in three Phi-
lippine villages. These interventions consisted of
improved water supply only, improved water supply
and waste disposal, and waste disposal only. Azurin
and Alvero (1974) found that the cholera disease
rate was reduced by 69 to 76 per cent but that there
was no marked difference in the effectiveness of the
three programs. This conclusion again points out
that an overall sanitary environment is necessary
before diseases such as cholera can be suppressed
entirely[37].

Health would also be improved if minimum stan-
dards would be respected in *housing*. It is reported
by Sharpston (1976) that better ventilated and larger houses would inhibit the spread of tuberculosis
and influenza. Note that one of the causes of bron-
chitis and lung diseases is the smoky and badly ventilated environment (due for instance to the location

of cooking fires inside the house) in which people may have to live. Spacier houses would also improve the health status of its inhabitants in the sense that diseases which are airborne are less likely to be transmitted.

1.3.4. EDUCATION

Earlier we have seen that the nutritional level is important to the health status of individuals. If education leads to better nutrition, education will *a fortiori* be an important variable in policies aiming at better health. Some evidence of a positive relationship between parental education and the nutritional level among children is given in Table 1.3. The positive relationship between education and nutrition can also be demonstrated by means of Table 1.4, where a comparison is made between the literacy among mothers of well nourished children on the one hand and mothers of malnourished children on the other hand. We can observe that the illiteracy rate is higher among mothers of malnourished children.

Cochrane *et.al.* (1980, pp.73-78) have also investigated the relationship between child mortality and mother's education for 17 Latin American and non-Latin American countries. In the regressions performed, the dependent variable was the probability of dying by age two (p_2) whereas the independent variable was numbers of years of school (YS). In almost all regressions the coefficients were statistically significantly different from zero. When the data for the seventeen countries were pooled, the following regression[38] equation was obtained:

$$p_2 = 0.114 - 0.009 \text{ YS} \qquad R^2 = 0.61$$

It appears therefore that, on average, an additional year of schooling of the mother decreases infant mortality by 9 per 1000. As an alternative, *the proportion of children dying, by age of mother,* was taken as the dependent variable to be regressed on YS. Here the same negative impact of YS on child mortality was found[39].

Note that Cochrane *et al.* (1980) also report on a fairly large number of multivariate studies that show the negative impact of parental education on child and infant mortality. In those studies, in-

Table 1.3. A comparison of average years of schooling of parents of malnourished and well
nourished children

Study	Sample size	Malnourished		Well nourished	
		Mothers years of school	Fathers years of school	Mothers years of school	Fathers years of school
Bogota,Colombia (Christiansen *et.al.*,1974)	181	2.9	3.1	3.9	4.5
Rural Mexico (Cravioto and Delicardie,1975)	38	1.9		2.1	
Santiago Chile (Selowsky and Taylor,1973)	39	3.7		3.8	
Kathmandu,Nepal (Graves,1978)	74	0.3	4.0	2.0	5.7
Iloilo, Philippines (Zeitlan and Formacion,1978)	68	3.8		4.5	
Weighted average		2.7	3.3	3.6	4.7

Source: Cochrane *et al.* (1980, p.65).

come is usually inserted in an equation as one of
the explanatory variables. The purpose is to try
to measure the *separate* effects of income and education. If education is the only explanatory variable of mortality or morbidity, there is indeed a
chance that its effect is overestimated since it
may capture part of the income effect. We will
mention briefly three of the most recent studies.
Firstly, from an analysis of data for 1294 women in
Managua (Nicaragua) in 1977, Behrman and Wolfe(1979)
found that infant mortality was reduced by 4 per
thousand by an additional year of mother's education.
Secondly, Schultz (1979) studied a sample of data
for 6692 urban women (age 30-34) and 3421 rural
women (age 30-34) in Colombia. For these age
groups he obtained statistically significant (nega-

tive) coefficients for the impact of wife's and
husband's literacy[40] on the *ratio of children dead
to children ever born*: for rural households, the
effect of both mother's and father's literacy was
-0.09, while for urban households the impact of
mother's literacy, -0.16, was twice that of father's
literacy. *Thirdly*, Anker and Knowles (1977) studied the impact of literacy rate upon mortality in
1969 in Kenya, by means of data on 41 districts.
It was found that the marginal effect of literacy
(in %) on infant and child mortality (in ‰) was
-0.80 and -0.20 respectively.

Table 1.4. A comparison of literacy between mothers
of malnourished and well nourished
children

Study	Sample size	Percent of illiterate mothers	
		Malnourished children	Well nourished children
Candelaria, Colombia (Wray & Aguirre,1969)	1094	34	29
Amman, Jordan (McLaren & Kanawati,1970)	611	84	72
Lebanon (Kanawati & McLaren,1973)	105	92	57
Punjab,India (Levinson,1974)	496	87	64
Average		61	49

Source: Cochrane *et al.* (1980, p.66).

1.3.5. TROPICAL DISEASE CONTROL

Control of the vector in vector-borne diseases seems
to be effective and comparatively inexpensive, but
there is the risk that after some time the parasite
and the vector become resistant to chemicals that
are used in vector control[41]. It is therefore necessary to have permanent monitoring of the disease

incidence[42]. Note that the WHO, the United Nations
Development Programme (UNDP) and the World Bank devote much effort to searching for effective control
measures in their *Special Programme for Research and
Training in Tropical Diseases.*

Evidence on the economic effects (*e.g.* the impact on labor supply) of diseases such as malaria,
filariasis and human trypanosomiasis is given in
Prescott (1979). An important study of the impact
of malaria on economic development has been written
by Conly (1975). Much interest has been directed to
the impact of malaria control (DDT spraying) on the
mortality rate and population growth rate in Sri
Lanka; Barlow (1967), Gray (1974), Meegema (1967,
1969) and Newman (1965, 1970, 1977) have contributed
to this particular topic. We only mention here the
most recent result by Newman (1977): he found by
means of regression analysis that 43.9 per cent of
the mortality decline in Sri Lanka between 1930 and
1960 due to malaria control.

1.3.6. RESULTS OF TWO PRIMARY HEALTH CARE INTER-
       VENTIONS

THE ETIMESGUT PROJECT IN TURKEY[43]

This project was initiated in 1966 by the Turkish
Ministry of Health, Hacettepe University and UNICEF
in order to 'provide integrated health and family
planning services in all areas of the (Etimesgut)
district, to establish training facilities for para-
medical personnel, and to conduct epidemiological
research relevant to rural health services and administration'[44]. The Etimesgut district is situated to the west of Ankara; it had a population of
55,000 in 1969. Particular problems in this area
where the contamination of village water supplies
and malnutrition; for instance, it was found that
between 15 and 29 per cent of preschoolers had insufficient calories and proteins.

In Figure 1.2 we present a picture of the components of the Etimesgut health structure. In Table
1.5 the responsibilities of the different agents of
this health system are described. One can clearly
see from Figure 1.2 and Table 1.5 that a *pyramidal*
structure of health care has been designed. *Firstly*, primary health services are provided as close
to the patients as possible,namely by the nurse-

Figure 1.2. Scheme of the health system in Etimesgut

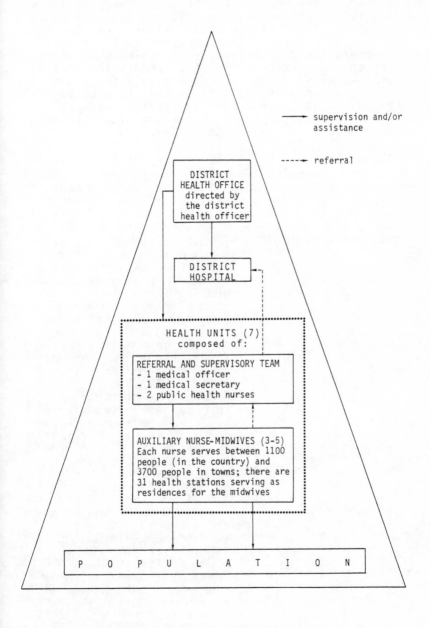

midwives. Only when a nurse-midwife judges that
she cannot treat a patient adequately, will she refer him to the medical officer. In turn the latter
will refer patients to the district hospital when
more specialized health personnel or treatment are
needed. *Secondly*, higher echelons in the health
structure are assisting or supervising the lower
echelons. In other words, they are at the service
of lower echelons who are responsible for the major-
ity of health services. It is thus recognized that
primary health care cannot be provided efficiently
if health services are directly organized by the
top echelons in the health system.

Table 1.5. Tasks of the agents in the Etimesgut
health care system

AGENT	TASKS
Health unit AUXILIARY NURSE-MIDWIFE	-scheduled immunization -family planning activities by means of in-home visits -in the case of pregnancy: scheduled examinations after the 4th month of pregnancy; supervising home birth; referring high risk pregnancy to medical officer or hospital; parents are given instruction on delivery when the nurse is not available at the time of birth -frequent home visits for each child (up to 6 years old), during which child care, nutrition and family planning are discussed -vaccination against TBC, whooping cough, tetanus toxoid, polio, smallpox, typhoid -monitoring of growth and development of children; referral to the medical officer in case of growth retardation -auxiliary nurse-midwives for rural areas have to reside in health stations -reporting all important events (pregnancy, birth, diseases etc.) and own activities to the medical officer

Table 1.5. (cont'd)

AGENT	TASKS
PUBLIC HEALTH NURSE	-female nurses: in-service train-ing and supervision of mothers in child care, family planning and provision of BCG vaccinations -male nurses: rural sanitation measures, school and male adult health education, communicable disease control, household census (twice yearly)
MEDICAL OFFICER	-examination of patients referred by nurse-midwives; referral to district hospital when needed -supervision of preventive and family planning activities -responsible for community health education and development -visits to health unit stations and villages to check data col-lected by nurse-midwives
District hospital	-provides a full range of curative services -to accept patients referred by medical officer
District health office	-health planning -training of professional staff

The health outcomes of this project are reported in Table 1.6.

Neonatal mortality in Etimesgut declined by 26 per cent over the period 1967 to 1977 whereas infant mortality declined by 50 per cent over the same pe-riod. Family planning activities were also effec-tive: the crude birth rate and the fertility rate declined by 24 per cent and 26 per cent respectively over the period 1967 to 1974. One can see that dur-ing the period 1967-1973, average infant mortality in Turkey also decreased, namely by 28 per cent. However, over that period the infant mortality rate in Etimesgut decreased faster, namely by 34 per cent. Gwatkin *et al*. (1980, p.52) warn, however, that 'with-

23

out data from an area socioeconomically comparable
to Etimesgut, it remains unclear whether the rural
health program was responsible for the faster decline in infant mortality'.

Table 1.6. Health outcomes of the primary health
care intervention in Etimesgut

Year	Etimesgut				Turkey infant mor- tality (‰)
	Neonatal mortality (‰) (0-30 days)	Infant mortality (‰) (1 month-1 year)	Crude birth rate (‰)	Total fertility rate	
1967	36.0	142.0	35.1	4.95	153.0
1968	39.3	121.0			
1969	28.5	111.0	35.4	4.94	
1970	25.7	103.2			
1971	32.5	87.6			
1972	30.2	112.0	29.5	3.97	
1973	34.3	93.1			110.0
1974	31.7	94.5	26.9	3.68	
1976	30.0	82.5			
1977	26.7	71.8	28.4		

Source: Gwatkin *et al.* (1980, p.17 and p.52).

THE JAMKHED PROJECT IN INDIA [4] [5]

This project, which started in 1971 in Jamkhed
(state of Maharashtra), is a comprehensive rural
health project that provides integrated curative,
preventive nutrition and health services. The specific aims of the project are the reduction of the
population growth rate, the morbidity and mortality
rates among the under-fives and the provision of
care for the chronically ill (especially those with
tuberculosis and leprosy).

The town of Jamkhed, that is situated 400 kilo-
meters southeast of Bombay, is part of the Ahmednagar
district, itself one of the poorest areas of the
state of Maharashtra. At the start of the project
thirty local villages around Jamkhed with a population of 40,000 people were part of the project.
Later on, in 1976, the number of villages and people
included in the project had doubled. Agricultural
production is the main activity in the Jamkhed area.

Before the project's start, health care was given by two physicians, ten auxiliary midwives and eight basic health workers. The main direct or associated cause of death of infants and young children was the malnutrition-diarrhea complex.

The structure of the project is depicted in Figure 1.3 whereas the tasks of the different categories of health agents are described in Table 1.7. The allocation of tasks shows that the health system has a *pyramidal* structure. Indeed, the basic health services and nutrition supplements are provided by village health workers and other community volunteers. Patients are only referred to the clinic and the hospital when there is a clear need for higher level care. In order to improve the access of the population to primary health care, special attention is paid to the selection of village health workers. They are usually middle-aged women that are chosen from three or four candidates by the community. The latter ensures that the village health workers are aware of their villages' health problems. This knowledge enables them better to adjust health services to the villages' needs.

Table 1.7. Tasks of the agents in the Jamkhed health care system

AGENT	TASKS
COMMUNITY VOLUNTEERS in charge of supplementary feeding program	Deserving under-fives receive one meal per day (50 grams of cereals, 20 grains pulses, 10 grams coarse sugar and 10 grams oil)
VILLAGE HEALTH WORKERS (VHW)	-identification and follow-up of pregnancies -supervision of home births -weighing and screening of under-fives for inadequate growth, diarrhea, fever, skin and eye infections -supervising of supplementary feeding program -collection of vital statistics -provision of simple health care and health education to villagers (includes child and maternal health care and family planning)

Table 1.7. (cont'd)

AGENT	TASKS
TWO MOBILE TEAMS	Provides weekly visits to project's villages
<u>Physician</u>	-training of VHW and mobile teams -together with the mobile team's social worker, he discusses with community leaders about the project's progress and the population's needs
<u>Paramedic</u>	In-home identification of tuberculosis and leprosy is a prime responsibility
<u>Nurse-Midwife</u>	-treats about 80 per cent of health problems seen -other patients are referred to the physician or the Jamkhed clinic -supervision of VHW and follow-up on all pregnant women identified by the VHW
JAMKHED CLINIC	-at the clinic training in maternal and child health and health education is given to VHW -accepts patients that are referred to the clinic by the VHW or the physician -X-ray and operating facilities are available to the patients
AHMEDNAGAR HOSPITAL	-accepts patients that cannot be treated at the Jamkhed clinic

In Table 1.8 some health outcomes of the project are presented. One notices that infant mortality has decreased substantially in the project area from 1971 to 1976. There is also a clear difference between infant mortality in the project and non-project areas in 1976. Family planning activities in the Jamkhed project have also resulted in a lower crude birth rate than in the non-project area. Some caution in interpreting the results is required, however, in the absence of significance tests or information on data collection and the socioeconomic characteristics of the project and non-project areas[46].

Figure 1.3. Scheme of the health system in the
Jamkhed project

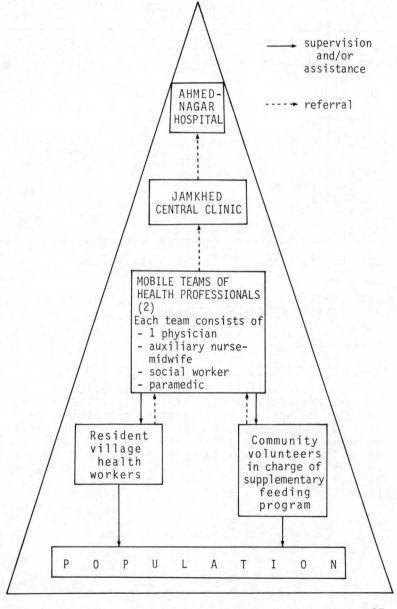

Table 1.8. Health outcomes of the primary health
care intervention in Jamkhed

Variables	Type of area		
	Project-area 1971	1976	Non-project area
Population surveyed	1,490	1,491	1,405
Immunization status of under-fives	less than 1 %	84 %	15 %
Infant mortality (deaths per 1000 live births)	97	39	90
Antenatal care	less than 0.5 % of all women	78 % of pregnant women	2 % of pregnant women
Percentage of eligible couples practicing contraception	2.5 %	50.5 %	10 %
Crude birth rate	40 ‰	23 ‰	37 ‰

Source: Gwatkin *et al.* (1980, p.17 and p.62).

1.4. EMPIRICAL EVIDENCE FROM MACRO-STUDIES[47] ON THE EFFECT OF HEALTH DETERMINANTS

1.4.1. THE WHEELER STUDY

Life expectancy at birth can be regarded as a suitable indicator for the health situation of the population. Since time series for life expectancy and
its determinants are generally unavailable for developing countries, cross-section regression analysis is usually used in order to measure the impact
of various health determinants. Wheeler (1980)
estimated a life expectancy equation, using data
for developing countries. Note that this equation
is part of a small basic needs growth model. His
result is the following[48] :

$$h = 0.099 + |0.171 - 0.028 \ln H_0| \; |q - p|$$
$$(0.015) \quad (0.436) \; (0.115)$$

$$+ \; |-0.320 + 0.085 \ln H_0 \; | \; d$$
$$(0.802) \; (0.208)$$

$$+ \; |-0.756 + 0.205 \ln H_0 \; | \; r$$
$$(0.614) \; (0.161)$$

$$+ \; | \; 3.140 - 0.803 \ln H_0 \; | \; n$$
$$(2.864) \; (0.724)$$

$$+ \; | \; 0.707 - 0.200 \ln H_0 \; | \; e \qquad R^2 = 0.27$$
$$(0.487) \; (0.134)$$

The variables written in small letters are all percentage changes from 1960-1970; they are defined as follows:

h   change in life expectancy at birth
q   change in gross domestic product
p   change in population
d   change in population per doctor
r   change in population per nursing person
n   change in per capita calories available
e   change in adult literacy rate.

The variable H_0 is the level of life expectancy at birth in 1960.

One can see that basic needs variables such as nutrition and education have positive impacts on life expectancy. Health services captured by the variables d and r also show beneficial effects upon life expectancy. The equation is specified in such a way that at initial low levels of life expectancy, the impact of a change in d, r, n and e is larger; in other words the effects of health determinants taper off as we approach higher life expectancy levels. There is also an income per capita variable in this equation in order to convey that as the population gets richer, more health improvements are made possible.

1.4.2. THE SHEEHAN-HOPKINS STUDY

Sheehan and Hopkins (1979) did a comprehensive study on basic needs performance and its determinants. In Table 1.9, we present selected results on the determinants of life expectancy, infant mortality and deaths due to infectious diseases. The latter two variables give additional information on the health status of the population. In the first three equations in Table 1.9 the impact of popula-

Table 1.9. Determinants of health status variables in the Sheehan and Hopkins study

Number of equation	Dependent variables	Explanatory variables							R^2
		Doctors per 100,000 people (1970)	Calorie consumption (1970)	Protein consumption (1970)	Access to water (1970)	GNP (1970)	Primary school enrolment (1970)	Population growth (1960-1970)	
(1)	Life expectancy (1970)					.68*** (65.6)		-.33*** (15.3)	.41
(2)	Infant mortality (1970)					-.59*** (34.5)		.21** (4.2)	.31
(3)	Deaths due to infectious diseases (1970)					-.68*** (25.0)		.72*** (28.3)	.64
(4)	Life expectancy (1970)					.34*** (16.4)	.48*** (33.3)		.50
(5)	Infant mortality (1970)					-.23*** (7.3)	-.63*** (53.8)		.58
(6)	Deaths due to infectious diseases (1970)					-.21 (1.0)	-.48*** (5.3)		.36
(7)	Life expectancy (1970)	.72*** (30.2)	.18 (2.1)	.19 (2.5)	.13 (1.6)	.01 (0.00)			.67
(8)	Infant mortality (1970)	-.41** (4.8)	-.14 (.62)	-.18 (1.0)	-.18 (1.5)	-.14 (.92)			.43

Source: Sheehan and Hopkins (1979, ch.5).

Note: - F values in parentheses (** = significance at 5 %, *** = significant at 1 %);
- all equations are linear;
- regression coefficients are beta weights (equal to the coefficient times the standard deviation of the corresponding variable divided by the standard deviation of the dependent variable).

tion growth and gross national product per capita
on health status is investigated. The coefficients
are all statistically significantly different from
zero. *First*, they reveal that population growth
has a negative impact on the health status of the
population. Note that in the third equation, population growth is as important as GNP in explaining
the variance of the death rate. *Secondly*, GNP also
has an important effect on the health status variables. One can think of GNP in these equations as
a proxy variable for health determinants such as
nutrition, water supply and sanitation, medical
personnel and education.

In equations (4) to (6), the effects of education, measured by the primary school enrolment
rate, and of GNP on health have been measured. We
again find significant coefficients. A major disadvantage of these equations is that other important
health determinants are not explicitly modeled.
In equations (7) and (8), an effort is made to measure the effects of these other health determinants.
To some extent, Sheehan and Hopkins were successful
in that all coefficients appear with the right sign.
However, they find that only the coefficient corresponding to the variable 'Doctors per 100,000 people' is statistically significantly different from
zero. Furthermore it is the variable that accounts
for most of the variance in life expectancy and infant mortality.

1.5. DESCRIPTIVE STATISTICS[49] OF HEALTH DETERMINANTS AND HEALTH STATUS, 1960-1980

The purpose of this section is to compare the health
determinants and health status of LDC in earlier
years (mainly 1960) with those in more recent years
(mainly 1980), and subsequently to draw some conclusions regarding health development in LDC. We will
also be able to verify, once again, the existence of
the relationships between health status and its various determinants. Note that the data pertain to 96
low and middle-income LDC and are collected from the
Statistical Appendix of various issues of the World
Bank's World Development Report. The data used are
listed in Appendix 2.

The *health determinants* studied are the percentage of population with access to safe water(ASW),
the population per physician (PHY), the population per

nurse (NUR), adult literacy in percentage terms (LIT),
daily per capita calorie supply as percentage of requirement (CAL), fertility rate (FERT) and the crude
birth rate per thousand population (CRB). The *health
status indicators* analyzed are the crude death rate
per thousand population (CRD), life expectancy at
birth in years (LIFE), the infant mortality rate of
children aged 0 to 1 year per thousand children (IM)
and the child death rate of children aged 1 to 4 per
thousand children (CD). The descriptive statistics
used are the mean, the variance and standard deviation, the coefficient of variation, the minimum, the
maximum, the range, the skewness and the kurtosis.
The descriptive statistics related to the health determinants and health status variables are presented
in Tables 1.10 and 1.11 respectively. Readers interested in the frequency distributions of these
variables are referred to Appendix 4.

Inspecting Table 1.10, one notices the drastic
change in the means of the variables PHY and NUR
over the period 1960-1977. The literacy rate, LIT,
has improved while the fertility rate, FERT, and the
crude birth rate, CRB, have decreased over time.
The relative dispersion, measured by the coefficient
of variation, has increased especially for NUR and
CRB. LIT is much less dispersed in 1977 than in
1966. The same type of skewness is maintained
through time. Yet, NUR is more skewed to the right
in 1977 than in 1960. The positive skewness of LIT
and CAL decreases while the skewness of FERT and CRB
becomes less negative. Note also that the kurtosis
of the distribution of NUR in 1977 reveals a well
pronounced narrowly shaped distribution. The kurtosis of the distributions of FERT and CRB becomes
negative in 1980, implying broadly shaped distributions.

The information in Table 1.10 clearly reveals
that the health determinants underwent a change that
was bound to be beneficial to health status. It can
indeed be verified in Table 1.11 that mortality
rates have decreased and that life expectancy has
increased. We notice, in addition, that the relative dispersion of the variables increases, except
for life expectancy. The skewness of the distributions of CRD and IM becomes positive in 1980. Also
note that for all health status variables the kurtosis remains negative over time.

Table 1.10. Descriptive Statistics of Health Determinants*

Indicator	Number of observations	Year	Mean	Variance	Standard deviation	Coefficient of variation	Minimum	Maximum	Range	Skewness	Kurtosis
ASW	70	1975	40.986	609.955	24.697	0.603	4	100	96	0.414	-0.981
PHY	85	1960	21626.700	9.093×10^8	30154.200	1.394	400	143290	142890	2.071	4.103
PHY	85	1977	11448.200	1.989×10^8	14103.800	1.232	310	74910	74600	1.967	4.343
NUR	66	1960	4392.800	1.611×10^7	4013.750	0.914	300	19590	19290	1.856	3.399
NUR	66	1977	2533.400	1.333×10^7	3650.960	1.441	250	25920	25670	4.422	24.136
LIT	63	1960	33.619	768.692	27.725	0.825	1	93	92	0.631	-0.969
LIT	63	1977	50.429	745.504	27.304	0.541	5	98	93	0.048	-1.275
CAL	95	1974	99.368	204.794	14.311	0.144	72	141	69	0.506	-0.039
CAL	95	1977	101.053	211.557	14.545	0.144	62	136	74	0.213	-0.093
FERT	95	1975	5.745	1.642	1.281	0.223	2.3	7.6	5.3	-1.161	0.585
FERT	95	1980	5.332	2.392	1.547	0.290	1.8	8.3	6.5	-0.572	-0.575
CRB	95	1960	44.305	57.238	7.566	0.171	19	55	36	-1.654	2.658
CRB	95	1980	38.505	103.934	10.195	0.265	16	56	40	-0.674	-0.526

* For the variables ASW, comparable data for years other than 1975 were not available.

Source: Own computations.

33

Table 1.11. Descriptive Statistics of Health Status

Indicator	Number of observations	Year	Mean	Variance	Standard deviation	Coefficient of variation	Minimum	Maximum	Range	Skewness	Kurtosis
CRD	95	1960	19.590	47.862	6.918	0.353	6	31	25	-0.237	-1.184
CRD	95	1980	13.390	32.921	5.738	0.429	5	26	21	0.303	-1.169
LIFE	94	1960	47.309	102.667	10.133	0.214	33	69	36	0.555	-0.862
LIFE	94	1980	55.968	106.293	10.310	0.184	37	74	37	0.085	-1.253
IM	94	1960	138.436	2663.920	51.613	0.373	32	252	220	-0.260	-0.741
IM	94	1980	94.883	2453.510	49.533	0.522	12	211	199	0.155	-0.734
CD	91	1960	28.110	242.477	15.572	0.554	2	63	61	0.025	-0.855
CD	91	1980	16.363	166.811	12.916	0.789	1	51	50	0.638	-0.342

Source: Own computations.

1.6. CONCLUDING REMARKS

We have demonstrated the need for an integrated basic needs approach to health care in developing
countries, by presenting and discussing evidence
about the major determinants of the health status
of people in LDC. One may wonder why income distribution and/or income growth were not discussed as
determinants of health. We recognize that they co-
determine health, but only indirectly. The reasoning is the following. Improvements in the health
determinants need to be financed out of governmental
budgets or out of private household income. It is
therefore evident that government's decision to allocate a certain percentage of total state expenditures to health care is crucial in planning health
improvements. Note that government's task of deciding between alternative allocations will become less
difficult if economic growth contributes to enlarg-
ing government's command of resources. Concerning
health care financing by households a vigorous
growth of GNP, together with a just income distribution, is an excellent way to increase the share of
income that households will allocate to health improving basic needs. Therefore, we consider income
distribution and income growth to be important elements in the *financing* of health determinants. For
a further treatment of the linkages between health
and economic development, the reader is referred to
the next chapter.

NOTES

[1] See World Bank (1982) Statistical Appendix.
These data are also presented in Appendix 2.
[2] See Morawetz (1977, p.43).
[3] Health services include for instance doctors'
and nurses' time inputs.
[4] Based to a large extent on World Bank (1980a)
and Kocher and Cash (1979).
[5] See World Bank (1980a), p.21.
[6] See Berelson *et al.* (1980) for a further discussion of the ingredients of population planning.
[7] See Appendix 1 for some data information
about the prevalence of malnutrition.
[8] See Winikoff and Brown (1980, pp.171-173).
[9] See Schneider *et al.* (1978, pp.2092-2093).
[10] *Ibidem.*
[11] See Mata (1978).
[12] See Appendix 1 for data about the prevalence

and mortality of major infections and parasitic diseases.

[13] For a description of the various tropical diseases, see Sterky (1977) and Wright and Baird (1971).

[14] See Schneider *et al.* (1978, pp.2092-2093).

[15] *Ibidem.*

[16] See World Bank (1980a, p.17); see also Djukanovic and Mach (1975, pp.8-9) and McEvers(1980, pp.48-49) on the objectives of primary health care. See Orubuloye and Oyeneye (1982) for a description of the primary health care systems in Nigeria, Sri Lanka and Tanzania.

[17] By micro-study we mean a study of health determinants in a specific community or city or in a specific group of households.

[18] Cited in Winikoff and Brown (1980, p.172).

[19] Cited in Mosley (1979, p.86).

[20] See Winikoff and Brown (1980, p.172).

[21] For a comprehensive study of the role of nutrition in development, see Berg, Scrimshaw and Call (1973).

[22] See Mosley (1979, p.86-87).

[23] See Kocher and Cash (1979).

[24] Also quoted in Kocher and Cash (1979, p.23).

[25] See Kocher and Cash (1979).

[26] See Chernichovsky (1979).

[27] See also Soysa (1981).

[28] See Sorkin (1976, p.31). See also Barlow (1979, pp.63-64) more evidence on the relation between malnutrition and children's health.

[29] See Clugston (1981, pp.34-36).

[30] *Ibidem.*

[31] See Kallen (1969), quoted in Wells and Klees (1980, p.13).

[32] See Clugston (1981, pp.36-37).

[33] See Wells and Klees (1980, p.13).

[34] See Curlin *et al.* (1977, p.14). For more information on the relation between health and water supply, see Briscoe (1978).

[35] See Van Zijl (1966, p.252).

[36] See Wagner and Lanoix (1958, p.22).

[37] See also World Bank (1976b, pp.54-57).

[38] See chapter 7 for an explanation of regression analysis.

[39] See Cochrane *et al.* (1980, p.77).

[40] Literacy is defined by Schultz as 3 years of schooling.

[41] See Walsh and Warren (1979).

[42] See World Bank (1980a, p.17).

[43] Based on Gwatkin *et al.* (1980, pp.50-52).

[44] Gwatkin *et al.* (1980, p.50).
[45] Based on Gwatkin *et al.* (1980, pp.59-62).
[46] See Gwatkin *et al.* (1980, p.62).
[47] By macro-studies we mean studies using aggregate data of countries.
[48] The figures beneath the coefficients are standard errors; the latter are explained in chapter 7.
[49] See Appendix 3 for a brief introduction to elementary descriptive statistics.

Chapter Two

ON THE LINKAGES BETWEEN HEALTH AND ECONOMIC
DEVELOPMENT

2.1. HEALTH AND ECONOMIC GROWTH: CAN BOTH BE
     ATTAINED SIMULTANEOUSLY?

There remains some uncertainty about the relation
between health improvements and economic growth.
Frequently it is reasoned that health improvements
are secured at the expense of investments in fixed
capital, entailing a smaller economic growth. A
study by Hicks (1980) suggests, however, that countries paying considerable attention to basic needs
certainly do not hold up economic growth. Indeed
the opposite is the case[1]. The reasoning here is
that basic needs policies lead to investments in
human capital that in turn are growth promoting. In
Tables 2.1 and 2.2 part of that evidence is reported.

        We first compare, in Table 2.1, life expectancy
and economic growth in the twelve fastest growing
countries for the period 1960-1977 (except oil ex-
porting countries and countries with populations
under one million). We see that those 12 countries
had a higher average life expectancy than the average
of all 83 countries studied by Hicks, namely 61 years
compared with 48 years. This suggests that health
status can even be a factor contributing to economic
growth. Hicks (1980, p.11) argues, however, that
the former comparison is biased, since the countries
with the highest growth rates were also those with
above average levels of income. He writes then that
it is no surprise that these fast growing countries
have above average life expectancy, since levels of
life expectancy and income are highly correlated.
He takes account of this bias in the following way:
he first estimates an equation explaining life expectancy by income; this allows him to calculate the
expected levels of life expectancy. Subsequently

the deviations from expected levels can be computed; these are indicators that are adjusted for the income level, of course. After comparing the deviations (column 3, Table 2.1) with the figures of economic growth, a conclusion identical to the above follows, *viz.* the existence of a positive relationship between health status and economic growth.

Table 2.1. Economic Growth and Life Expectancy, selected countries

Country	Average Growth Rate of Real GNP (%) 1960-1977	Life Expectancy at birth (in years) 1960	Deviations from Expected Levels of Life Expectancy (in years) 1960
Singapore	7.7	64	3.1
Korea	7.6	54	11.1
Taiwan	6.5	64	15.5
Hong Kong	6.3	65	6.5
Greece	6.1	68	5.7
Portugal	5.7	62	4.7
Spain	5.3	68	1.8
Yugoslavia	5.2	62	4.7
Brazil	4.9	57	3.0
Israel	4.6	69	2.0
Thailand	4.5	51	9.5
Tunisia	4.3	48	-0.5
Average: Top 12	5.7	61	5.6
Average: 83 countries	2.4	48	0.0

Note: Expected or normal levels of life expectancy were estimated using a regression equation in which per capita income and per capita income squared featured as explanatory variables.

Source: Hicks (1980, p.12).

It is important to realize that this positive relationship between health and economic growth does not prove that health development is a sufficient condition for economic growth. Indeed, it would be dangerous to say that a better health status always leads to higher growth. To investigate the latter problem, Hicks studied the growth rates of the

twelve countries with the highest deviation from expected levels of life expectancy. One is referred
to Table 2.2 for this comparison. It can be noticed
that countries such as Burma, Kenya, Paraguay and
the Philippines who did well in terms of life expectancy did not have very high growth rates. Still,
an interesting fact is that the average growth rate
of those countries, i.e. 4 per cent, is higher than
the group average of 2.4 per cent. In other words
countries who did well in terms of health status
also had a better than average record in terms of
economic growth. Although Hicks' study is quite
interesting, it does not provide a comprehensive
treatment of the mechanism of the linkages between
health and economic growth. The latter is surely
not an easy phenomenon to grasp since economic
growth depends, directly and indirectly, upon a
large number of economic as well as non-economic
variables. To think that health improvement would
in all circumstances trigger a higher growth rate
would be naive. However, considering the empirical
evidence just studied, we may claim at least that
there does not have to be a contradiction between
health improvement and economic growth.

Table 2.2. Economic Growth and Life Expectancy,
selected countries

Country	Deviations from Expected Levels of Life Expectancy (in years) 1960	Average Growth Rate of Real GNP (%) 1960-1977
Sri Lanka	22.5	1.9
Taiwan	15.5	6.5
Korea	11.1	7.6
Thailand	9.5	4.5
Malaysia	7.3	4.0
Paraguay	6.9	2.4
Philippines	6.8	2.1
Hong Kong	6.5	6.3
Panama	6.1	3.7
Burma	6.0	0.9
Greece	5.7	6.1
Kenya	5.5	2.4
Average 12 countries	9.1	4.0
Average 83 countries	0.0	2.4

Note: See Table 2.1.

Source: Hicks (1980, p.16).

2.2. A MODEL OF LINKAGES BETWEEN HEALTH AND ECONOMY

2.2.1. INTRODUCTION

Section 1.5 above gave some empirical information about the evolution during the past decades of a number of health indicators. It could be seen that the health status indicators underwent a change that is parallel to that of the health determinants. At the same time the economies of countries with a higher than average life expectancy also grew faster than the average developing country. Although we know that health and economic growth do not have to be enemies, we still are confronted with the question of what is the precise role of economic development in health improvement and vice versa. The answer to this question is likely to be very complex. The latter explains partly why the empirical research in this area is very much limited. We will try here to elucidate this issue by studying a fairly simple prototype model of the linkages between health and economic development. We still first present the structure of the model and discuss the various linkages afterwards.

2.2.2. STRUCTURE OF THE MODEL

In order to keep the model as simple as possible, we envisage an economy with two sectors, namely the food and non-food sector. There will be three main blocks in the model, dealing with, consecutively, the economy at large, primary health care expenditures and health indicators. Before studying the mathematical structure of the model, the reader is asked to inspect first the model's diagram; see Figure 2.1 on page 43. The symbols used in that diagram are explained in Table 2.3. The effects going from one variable to another are represented in the diagram by arrows, each arrow carrying a number which will be referred to in the discussion of the model's linkages.

Table 2.3. Explanation of symbols

Symbol	Explanation
BC	Birth control measures
CAF	Utilization of capital in food sector
CANF	Utilization of capital in non-food sector
CD	Infant and child mortality age 0-4
CF	Capital in food sector
CNF	Capital in non-food sector
CRB	Birth rate
CRD	Mortality above age 4
CUR	Curative services
DEB	Debility
DFC	Demand for food per capita
EDUC	Health education
EI	Income of enterprises
FAC	Food availability per capita
FPR	Food prices
GI	Government income
HI	Household income
HIC	Household income per capita
L	Labor
LF	Labor in food sector
LNF	Labor in non-food sector
LQF	Quality of labor in food sector
LQNF	Quality of labor in non-food sector
MAL	Degree of malnutrition
MF	Food imports
MFRC	Minimum food requirements per capita
MORB	Morbidity
NI	National income
NUTRI	Nutrition intervention
PARA	Parasitic disease control
PF	Production of food
PGR	Population growth
PNF	Production of non-food
POP	Population
RFC	Real food consumption per capita
SAN	Improvements in sanitary conditions

We now present the model's relationships in a mathematical form: such a format has the advantage that one has a clear view of the determinants of each health or economic variable that is to be explained. The sign under an explanatory variable gives the direction (positive or negative) of the likely impact upon the dependent variable[2]. The symbol f refers to *function*. Note also that the

Figure 2.1. Linkages between health and the economy

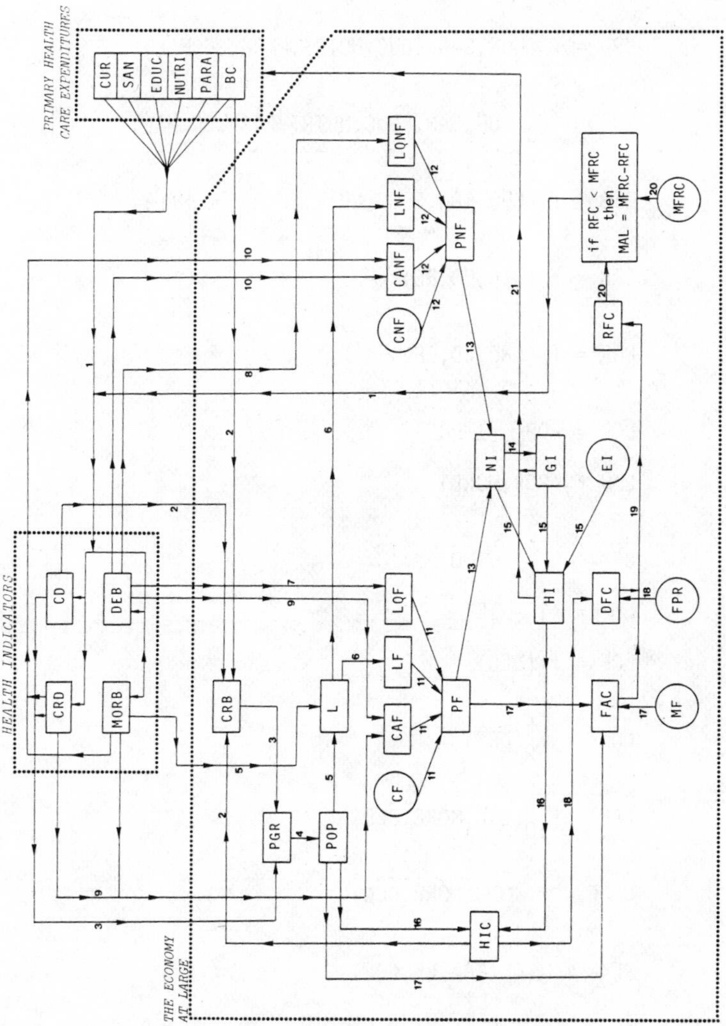

43

number after each equation refers to the arrow with the corresponding number in the diagram. The equations are the following[3]:

$$CRD = f_1(\underset{-}{CUR},\underset{-}{SAN},\underset{-}{EDUC},\underset{-}{NUTRI},\underset{-}{PARA},\underset{-}{BC},\underset{+}{MAL}) \tag{1}$$

$$CD = f_2(\underset{-}{CUR},\underset{-}{SAN},\underset{-}{EDUC},\underset{-}{NUTRI},\underset{-}{PARA},\underset{-}{BC},\underset{+}{MAL}) \tag{1}$$

$$MORB = f_3(\underset{-}{CUR},\underset{-}{SAN},\underset{-}{EDUC},\underset{-}{NUTRI},\underset{-}{PARA},\underset{-}{BC},\underset{+}{MAL}) \tag{1}$$

$$DEB = f_4(\underset{-}{CUR},\underset{-}{SAN},\underset{-}{EDUC},\underset{-}{NUTRI},\underset{-}{PARA},\underset{-}{BC},\underset{+}{MAL}) \tag{1}$$

$$CRB = f_5(\underset{-}{HIC},\underset{+}{CD},\underset{-}{BC}) \tag{2}$$

$$PGR = f_6(\underset{-}{CRD},\underset{-}{CD},\underset{+}{CRB}) \tag{3}$$

$$POP = POP_{-1}(1+PGR) \tag{4}$$

$$L = f_7(\underset{+}{POP},\underset{-}{MORB}) \tag{5}$$

$$LF = \alpha L \qquad \alpha > 0 \tag{6}$$

$$LNF = (1-\alpha)L \tag{6}$$

$$LQF = f_8(\underset{-}{DEB}) \tag{7}$$

$$LQNF = f_9(\underset{-}{DEB}) \tag{8}$$

$$CAF = f_{10}(\underset{-}{CRD},\underset{-}{MORB},\underset{-}{DEB}) \tag{9}$$

$$CANF = f_{11}(\underset{-}{CRD},\underset{-}{MORB},\underset{-}{DEB}) \tag{10}$$

$$PF = f_{12}(\underset{+}{CF},\underset{+}{CAF},\underset{+}{LF},\underset{+}{LQF}) \tag{11}$$

$$PNF = f_{13}(\underset{+}{CNF},\underset{+}{CANF},\underset{+}{LNF},\underset{+}{LQNF}) \tag{12}$$

$$NI = PF + PNF \tag{13}$$

$$GI = \tau NI \tag{14}$$

$$HI = NI - GI - EI \tag{15}$$

$$HIC = HI/POP \tag{16}$$

$$FAC = (PF + MF)/POP \tag{17}$$

$$DFC = f_{14}(\underset{+}{HIC}, \underset{-}{FPR}) \tag{18}$$

$$RFC = Min(DFC, FAC) \tag{19}$$

If RFC < MFRC, then
$$MAL = MFRC - RFC \tag{20}$$

$$CUR = f_{15}(\underset{+}{GI}, \underset{+}{HI}) \tag{21}$$

$$SAN = f_{16}(\underset{+}{GI}, \underset{+}{HI}) \tag{21}$$

$$EDUC = f_{17}(\underset{+}{GI}, \underset{+}{HI}) \tag{21}$$

$$NUTRI = f_{18}(\underset{+}{GI}, \underset{+}{HI}) \tag{21}$$

$$PARA = f_{19}(\underset{+}{GI}, \underset{+}{HI}) \tag{21}$$

$$BC = f_{20}(\underset{+}{GI}, \underset{+}{HI}) \tag{21}$$

2.2.3. COMMENTS ON THE LINKAGES[4]

The first relationships in the model (a1) concern the linkages between primary health care intervention and the health indicators crude death rate, infant and child mortality, morbidity and debility. These interventions have a positive influence on health status, as demonstrated in the first chapter. Hence, they have a negative effect on the retained health indicators. Malnutrition aggravates the health problems and has therefore a positive effect upon mortality, morbidity and debility.

The birth rate is supposed to be influenced primarily by household income per capita, infant and child mortality and birth control measures (a2). Income has a negative effect on the crude birth rate, conveying that increasing individual welfare is likely to have a depressing effect upon the demand for children. Infant and child mortality have a positive effect on the crude birth rate. One can explain this by the fact that many parents in developing countries try to compensate for the eventual early death of their children by a high fertility rate. Hence, the lower infant and child mortality, the lower the birth rate is presumed to be.

Population growth (a3) obviously depends on the mortality and birth rates. In turn population growth determines population (a4). The amount of workers in man-years will be determined by the population size and the morbidity level (a5). The labor force in the food and non-food sector is then derived from the total labor force (a6).

Debility, that measures the productive capacity of the workers, influence the quality of the labor force in both sectors (a7 and a8). The utilization of capital in a developing economy is often influenced, not only by the state of the economy[5], but also by the health status of the population (a9 and a10). This is especially applicable in rural areas, where fertile soil is insufficiently exploited due, for instance, to epidemics of malaria. McEvers mentions[6] that 'when a disease as malaria has been brought under control, as in the Terai Hills of Nepal and India, rice growing areas of Sri Lanka or the canal area of Panama, major advances have apparently been made possible in agriculture and other resource developments'. Furthermore, it is known that diseases such as trypanosomiasis and onchocerciasis have caused abandonment of fertile land!

Production in both sectors is determined by capital, the amount of labor and labor quality (a11 and a12). National income is derived by adding production in the food and non-food sector (a13). By applying a constant tax rate τ to national income, government income is derived (a14). Household income is obtained by subtracting enterprise and government income from national income (a15). Household income and population lead subsequently to household income per capita(a16).

Food availability per capita is equal to the sum of food production and imports divided by population (a17). The demand for food per capita is determined by household income per capita and food prices (a18). The concept of real food consumption per capita is then introduced in order to convey that demand for food cannot always be met. It is equal to the minimum of the demand for food per capita and food availability per capita (a19). In other words if demand for food exceeds food availability, real food consumption will necessarily be equal to food availability. If real food consumption is smaller than the minimum food requirements for a healthy life, malnutrition will arise; the latter is measured by the difference between minimum food requirements and real food consumption (a20). Finally, it is specified that part of government income and of household income is used to finance primary health care expenditures (a21).

2.2.4. MAIN PROPOSITIONS FOLLOWING FROM THE MODEL

First, health services are financed by government and household income. The latter variables are determined within the model. Note that in the model government income is linked to national income by means of a constant rate of taxation. The higher the national income, the higher therefore government income and the amount of funds that can be allocated to primary health care services. Furthermore, if national income grows, household income is likely to increase, resulting in larger private expenditures for health care. Thus, economic growth can help to realize health objectives in an indirect way.

Secondly, if health status improves, the quantity and quality of labor and the utilization of capital are likely to be increased. Indeed, a healthy worker will probably work more and better than a sick person. In addition a healthy working population tends to make a better use of the existing capital stock. These increases in inputs will lead to a higher national production that in turn will contribute, as described above, to a better health status.

Thirdly, malnutrition is included as a determinant in the health indicator equations. One may show that the positive impact of primary health care policies on health status can be mitigated or annihilated by inadequate food policies. Indeed, consider the following scenario: due to increased health interventions, mortality rates are likely to decrease. The latter increase population growth, *cet.par.*, and stimulate the overall demand for food. If food production is inadequate and if, simultaneously, imports are limited (due to balance of payments problems, say), malnutrition may arise and may wipe out the temporary gains of health interventions. Government can then search for policies that reduce the malnutrition: food prices can be manipulated, labor and capital can be allocated to agricultural production or more food can be imported.

Fourthly, the scenario just described assumes the birth rate to be constant. Of course, one may hope that the fertility rate will respond to a declining infant and child mortality rate. Yet, one often reads in the health literature that, together with a decline in infant and child mortality, a certain level of economic development must be attained before fertility starts to drop[7]. This idea is somehow incorporated in the prototype model: the equation explaining the crude birth rate reveals that if there is a decline in household income, the effects of a decreasing infant and child mortality rate on the birth rate may be eliminated.

2.3. CONCLUDING REMARKS

The model above intends to indicate that there are many direct as well as indirect links between health and economic variables. It reveals that there are several instruments that governments can use to increase the health status in their countries. The principal policy instruments are, in this model, the rate of taxation (a14) and the allocation of government funds to primary health care expenditures (a21). We have also argued above that food production was important in guaranteeing a healthy life. Government and private households can work towards the goal of adequate food supply by allocating sufficient labor to the agricultural sector (a6). In addition the size of the capital stock in the food sector is an important instrument in enhancing food supply (a11).

It is evident that the model can be generalized by introducing additional economic sectors, demographic characteristics of the population, the income distribution, epidemiological factors etc. The model can also be made more dynamic, *viz*. the lags in the effects between variables can be modeled more explicitly. The model also needs to be filled with important variables that are specific to the economy that is modeled. A final remark is in order about the size of the economy modeled. We think that the model can be used as a starting point for a macro-economic analysis, *viz.* pertaining to the economy of a country as a whole, as well as for a micro-economic analysis, related to the economy of a province, region or even a village. It also goes without saying that the model needs to be given em-pirical content before it can effectively be used in the process of understanding the links between health and the economy in a specific environment.

NOTES

[1] See also Streeten (1981).
[2] See chapter 7 for an introduction to the estimation of mathematical equations.
[3] In the equation explaining population, -1 refers to a one year-lag.
[4] In this subsection a1 has to be read as 'arrow 1' in the diagram, *etc.*
[5] Its influence will be ignored here for sim-plicity's sake.
[6] See McEvers (1980, p.45).
[7] See *e.g. Ibidem* (pp.42-43).

PART II

METHODS FOR ECONOMIC EVALUATION   IN HEALTH CARE

Chapter Three

COST-BENEFIT ANALYSIS

3.1. DEFINITION

We will define cost-benefit analysis (CBA) as an approach to measure benefits and costs to *society* of a project or of a series of projects. The basic proposition is that benefits of a project should outweigh its costs if that project is to be accepted. If a choice has to be made between several alternative projects, the project with the greatest net benefit has to be chosen. Note that both benefits and costs are measured in terms of money.

3.2. MEASUREMENT OF BENEFITS AND COSTS

The most refined and correct way to measure a project's *benefits* is to find out which is the maximum amount that *society* is willing to pay for that project. The latter represents the gross welfare gain to society. Society's willingness to pay (WTP) is, in principle, equal to the sum of individuals' WTP. The concept of an individual's WTP will be further explained by means of the following example. Suppose that a particular health project provides a certain type of medical care to individuals. Neoclassical demand theory then defines a *demand curve* for each individual indicating the relationship between the price (p_m) and the desired quantity of medical care (q_m). This relationship is negative conveying that as p_m diminishes, q_m rises; see Figure 3.1. Imagine that government provides quantity OA. Demand theory says that, at the amount OA, the marginal utility of medical care is equal to AB^1. Moreover for all intramarginal units of medical care, the marginal utility is indicated by the demand curve[2]. For instance, at OE the marginal utility

of medical care is EF, at OC the marginal utility is
CD *etc*. It follows that the utility of OA is represented by the area under the demand curve between
O and A, namely OGBA. Suppose now that the individual actually pays OHBA for the amount OA. The area
GHB is then called *consumer's surplus*. In other
words the individual's WTP is equal to the effective
payment OHBA plus consumer's surplus GHB.

Figure 3.1. Demand for medical care by an individual

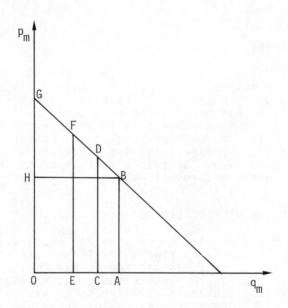

As was said above, society's WTP equals the sum
of the individual's WTP. This implies that society
attaches the same value to each individual's WTP.
It is a strong hypothesis that needs to be modified
whenever government intends to introduce distributional considerations into the CBA.

In CBA the *true cost* of a particular project
is the *opportunity cost* or the value of the benefits
one sacrifices if resources are not used in a rival
project. In other words, costs are the foregone
benefits of the next best project. Applied to
health projects, this means that if one uses health

personnel and drugs as inputs for a project, one has to inquire into the benefits these health resources would produce in the next best health project. Sometimes the next best alternative is not defined, however. In that case one usually puts the opportunity cost equal to the foregone benefits of allocating the inputs into the economy at large. Usually, one makes use of marginal productivity schedules of the inputs to obtain a measure of the benefits these inputs entail. Indeed, these schedules indicate the maximum amount that society is willing to pay for these inputs.

The net welfare gain or *net value* of a project $x(NV_x)$ is now equal to

$$NV_x = WTP_x - WTP_y,$$

where y refers to the next best alternative project. If the latter is not or cannot be defined

$$NV_x = WTP_x - WTP_x^i,$$

where WTP_x^i refers to society's WTP for the inputs used alternatively in the economy at large. If NV_x is positive, the project x may be undertaken. When several projects compete with each other, it is evident that the one with the highest NV needs to be selected in order to maximize welfare.

Up to now, we have given some basic elements of CBA for projects that have benefits or costs in the current period. It is evident that projects may also entail future benefits and future costs. Some modification in the calculation of net value will be required in this case. Note that it is generally accepted that individuals prefer a net value of 1 $ now to 1 $ received in the future. In other words 1 $ now and 1 $ one year hence will not have the same value. It follows that one can not simply add up benefits or costs that are related to different points in time. A *social discount rate*, denoted as r, will enable us to add up a stream of net benefits. Namely, 1 $ in year one will be worth $(1+r)$ $ in year two, $(1+r)^2$ $ in year three *etc*. Conversely, 1 $ in year two is worth $(1/1+r)$ $ in year one, 1 $ in year three is worth $(1/1+r)^2$ $ in year one *etc*. The value in year one of a $ received or paid in the future is called the present value of that dollar. Making use of the social discount rate r, we can calculate the *net present value* (NPV) of a project

$$NPV = \sum_{t=1}^{T} \frac{B_t - C_t}{(1+r)^{t-1}} \qquad (3.1)$$

where B and C refer to benefits and costs respectively while t is the time index. In fact, B_t is equal to the WTP for the project at time t while C_t has to be understood as the benefits foregone in period t. Note that if NPV > 0 society's welfare will increase, hence the project can be adopted. Again, if several projects are competing with each other, the one with the highest NPV should be chosen.

3.3. PROBLEMS IN BENEFIT MEASUREMENT

When evaluating benefits of a health intervention one should pay considerable attention to its real output. Above, in order to explain the WTP approach, the example was given of a health project that provided a certain type of medical care. The latter can only be considered as an approximation of that project's output, since the real output is the *improvement in health status*. Measures of this health status improvement involve primarily mortality and morbidity rates. The correct way to calculate the monetary benefit of a health status improvement, prescribed by economic theory, is to calculate how much society is willing to pay for that improvement.

In some studies we find the application of the willingness-to-pay-approach. Let us cite that, by estimating individuals' WTP for a reduction in the probability of dying, Acton (1975) is able to show that society is willing to pay a certain amount of money to reduce the occurence of heart and circulatory diseases. Jones-Lee (1976) uses a similar approach in order to estimate the value of safety. These studies are exceptions, however. There are several reasons for the lack of application of the WTP approach. *First*, when relying on the WTP approach, one trusts that the individual is able to make a correct assessment of the expected health status improvement. Frequently policy-makers and planners question this so-called consumer sovereignty by positing that the individual often misjudges the correct health status changes. The latter would be an argument against WTP estimation by means of a questionnaire. *Secondly*, in many developing coun-

tries a number of health interventions are introduced for the first time, hence one cannot make use
of empirically observed demand curves to calculate
the WTP. *Thirdly,* if individuals' WTP can be solic-
ited, one may voice objection against the fact that
the answers are linked to the existing income distribution. If the WTP are subsequently added in the
benefit calculation, one attaches implicitly more
importance to high income receivers with, presum-
ably, a high WTP than to low income receivers with
a low WTP. *Fourthly,* in a number of health interventions the major benefit consists of averted death.
In those cases it would be awkward to ask people
what they are willing to pay to avert a certain
death, since the value of life to a person is likely
to be almost infinitely high when he is confronted
with the choice between life and death[3].

A major alternative to the WTP approach is to
consider the benefits of a project as consisting of
the value of *production gained* and/or the *cost savings* as a result of that project. The gain of production can be the consequence of a decrease in mortality, morbidity (loss of working time) and debility (loss of productive capacity while at work)[4]. It
is frequently estimated by using earnings data pertaining to the individuals whose health has improved.
The cost savings can also be regarded upon as benefits because the funds freed by a project can finance other benefit entailing health projects. Several problems may arise while using this alternative, however. *First,* it is not sure that one can
simply use the wage rate of workers as a measure of
the gain in production. If one uses a wage rate
that happens to be set artificially above workers'
marginal productivity, the gross value of a project
will be overestimated. One therefore has to use the
shadow wage rate, viz. the wage rate that correctly
reflects workers' productivity. *Secondly,* suppose
that there are women, children, handicapped and old
aged among the beneficiaries of a project. How is
their contribution to society's product to be measured? Production benefits of health improvements
for women can be calculated by making use of the
wages women earn or can earn in the labor market.
In order to measure the benefits of health improvements for children one has to calculate their contribution to society's future output. Health care
for the old aged or handicapped may have no immedi-
ate economic benefit. Yet, society may,in any case,
attach a certain value to the health care for the

so-called unproductive. One comes to the conclusion that in such cases one should ideally use the
WTP approach! *Thirdly*, if cost savings are actually
used in the benefit calculation, there is a chance
that total benefits will be underestimated: indeed
the additional health interventions that can be financed by those freed funds may result in benefits
that exceed these interventions' financial cost.
Fourthly, this alternative approach is sometimes
attacked for its lack of consideration for *intangible benefits* such as reduction of pain and misery.
One forgets, however, that a possible omission of
intangible benefits is precisely the result of not
using the WTP approach!

To summarize, we must recognize that the WTP
approach provides a theoretically sound way to calculate health benefits in monetary terms. Yet given
the problems mentioned above, one can understand why
health researchers prefer alternatively methods. In
any event, it would certainly not be wise to auto-
matically discard the WTP approach. In addition,
one must always bear in mind that gain of production
and cost savings merely constitute an *approximation*
to the true welfare benefits.

3.4. PROBLEMS IN COST MEASUREMENT

We have already emphasized the necessity to view a
project's costs as the foregone benefits of the best
alternative project. If a project is not competing
in particular with another project, one needs to
calculate the benefits foregone by withdrawing inputs from the economy at large. Society's willingness to pay for an input will indicate the benefit
generated by that input. In the case of labor inputs (*e.g.* health workers, nurses, physicians), one
generally approximates WTP by the earnings of the
relevant skill category. However, the latter will
only reflect true social productivity if labor markets are competitive and if the project involves
only small movements of labor from one sector of the
economy to another. *First*, competitiveness of labor
markets signifies that all labor can be hired at the
prevailing market wage and that the users of labor
do not exercise any monopoly buying power in the
labor market. These conditions lead to an equality
between the market wage rate and the value of marginal productivity[5], hence the market wage can be
used to measure the loss to society of withdrawing

a unit of labor from the economy at large. *Secondly,* only if the project is small can the market wage be used as a measure of the marginal productivity for all units of labor. Indeed, large projects entail such a withdrawal of resources that marginal productivity will not remain constant. In that case one needs to know the demand curve[6] for labor in order to measure the total production loss caused by the withdrawn resources. Note further that when non-human inputs (such as drugs, hospital buildings *etc.*), are involved in a project, one should also proceed by estimating society's WTP for these inputs.

When input markets are non-competitive, one needs to estimate the *shadow prices* of the inputs, *viz.* the prices that correctly express the inputs' social productivity. A special issue arises when inputs have to be *imported*. These may cause a decrease in the foreign exchange available for other uses. One then needs to estimate the willingness to pay for this foreign exchange or its shadow price. Only in competitive foreign exchange markets will the official exchange rate reflect this willingness to pay. In the case of restrictions in the foreign exchange market, the willingness to pay is usually higher than the official exchange rate. Note also that when imported inputs are financed by grants, the opportunity cost will be zero if inputs are project specific or if there is no reduction of grants to other feasible projects. When projects are financed by loans, the repayments do of course entail a cost in terms of foreign exchange foregone.

3.5. SOME REFINEMENTS IN COST-BENEFIT ANALYSIS

3.5.1. THE APPROPRIATE SOCIAL DISCOUNT RATE

Above we stated that individuals' preferences for the present *vis-à-vis* the future is the reason why future benefits and costs are to be discounted. Individuals are likely to have such a preference because they expect to reach higher levels of consumption in the future; it may be accepted that as the level of consumption increases, the marginal utility of additional consumption will decrease. In other words the gain in net benefits in the future may be valued less than an identical gain in the present. One may therefore attach weights to aggregate net benefits such that they decline in time; for instance, when we designate the present net benefit as the unit of account, we can write the aggregate net benefits for a project that lasts T years as

$$\sum_{t=1}^{T} v_t(B_t - C_t) \qquad (3.2)$$

where v_1 is fixed at 1 and where the weights $v_2,\ldots,$ v_T decline over time. Let us now express the social discount rate r as the constant rate at which the weights on net benefits decline over time. It can then be shown[7] that (3.2) reduces exactly to the formula for the net present value (NPV) given above in (3.1). A major line of thought is to view the social discount rate r as a parameter that depends upon the *value judgments* of the cost-benefit analysts. In other words r would depend upon the analysts' judgment of the value of future gains *versus* the value of present gains to society. Namely the higher (lower) the social discount rate the more (less) the weights that are given to society's future gains will decline over time.

The above procedure may seem a little arbitrary since there is no objective measure of the social discount rate. Sometimes, therefore, the use is advocated of the *social opportunity cost* of public investment in health projects as the appropriate discount rate. The reasoning is the following. If funds are not invested in the public sector, it is very likely that they are invested in the private sector. The rate of return that is earned in the private sector can now be selected as the discount rate. Public projects are expected to incorporate at least that particular rate of return. If we, therefore, use this rate of return as the discount rate, the decision rule becomes the following: if the net present value is positive, the project should certainly be adopted since the public project gives a higher amount of welfare to society than the private project; if the net present value is negative the public project is worse than the private project.

This approach has also its disadvantages. *First*, it is possible that public funds have no alternative use in the private sector because of slack in the economy. *Secondly*, it is not that simple to pinpoint a single private rate of return since the latter may depend upon the type of industry with which the alternative private project is associated.

We see that there remains some uncertainty about the selection of the optimal discount rate[8]. However, Feldstein (1972) has argued that it is definitely inappropriate to select the social opportunity cost of public investment as the social discount rate. The reason is that one takes account already of alternative opportunities in the private sector while computing the costs in CBA. One therefore generally counsels to adopt the first approach outlined above, that is to view the social discount rate as a parameter that is specified according to the value judgments of the cost-benefit analysts. It is evident that the decision-makers will have to be fully aware of the implied values and the consequences of selecting a particular value for the social discount rate.

3.5.2. DISTRIBUTION WEIGHTS

When individuals' net benefits resulting from a project are added, it is implied that each unit of benefit has the same welfare significance. Indeed, in that case, the net benefit of 1 $ to a rich individual has the same value to society as the net benefit of 1 $ to a poorer individual. It is possible now that society wants to incorporate distributional objectives into the CBA. For instance, in health projects one may want to attach a greater *distribution weight* to the net benefits accruing to low income receivers than to those enjoyed by high income receivers. This does not have to mean that one considers the health status of the former to be more important than that of the latter. It generally implies that the monetary equivalent of an *improvement* in health status for the poor is valued more by society than that of the richer categories.

Various possibilities[9] are available to estimate the distribution weights. First, one could derive values for the distribution weights that are implicit in past government decisions concerning the distribution of benefits. Another method consists of using as weights the inverse of the marginal income tax rates applicable to the income groups considered; if income taxes are progressive, this method means that one weights the net gains to lower-income groups more heavily than the net gains of the higher-income groups. Lastly, one could use the ratio of the national income per capita to the average income of a particular income group as a weight for the net benefits of that income group. The latter will also tilt distribution weights in favor of lower-income groups.

3.5.3. RISKY PROJECTS

It has to be granted that projects often entail benefits and costs whose magnitude depends upon the occurrence of a number of events. We can then say that these benefits and costs are *risky*. In health interventions, events have to be understood as different states of the world that produce different health outcomes. For instance, an anti-parasitic disease campaign may lead to different degrees of effectiveness each associated with some probability.

If one knows the probability distribution of the states of the world, one can adjust the decision rule. Suppose that we consider a health intervention resulting in 10 alternative sequences of events with their corresponding net gains. Each sequence of events is associated with a particular probability p^i. Formula (3.1) can be adjusted in order to give the *expected net present value* (ENPV):

$$ENPV = \sum_{i=1}^{10} p^i \sum_{t=1}^{T} \frac{B_t^i - C_t^i}{(1+r)^{t-1}}$$

where the superscript i refers to the sequence of events i. Remember also that the sum of the p^i has to be equal to 1.

3.5.4. INDIRECT EFFECTS

In CBA one often attaches importance, in the first place, to the net gains for a project's target population. However, in many cases a project has also an impact on individuals (producers and consumers) outside the project. These impacts are called *indirect or external effects*. For instance, a health project comprising the eradication of the simulium fly (the vector of river blindness) may make certain fertile but abandoned lands (due to the illness) fully accessible again to the *whole* population. This health project would then not only generate benefits in terms of health status improvement but also in terms of additional production possibilities for society as a whole. If the WTP approach to benefit evaluation is used, there is a chance that if people are well informed, these indirect benefits are reflected by the willingness to pay. If the alternative approach is used, one has to check carefully whether such indirect but important benefits are not overlooked.

Another example of indirect effects is the following. Suppose that a health intervention program consists of improving the nutritional status of children. The method adopted to enhance children's nutrition is to give nutrition education to mothers. The direct benefits would consist of children's health benefits. Yet *indirect benefits* are likely to consist of improved health of the mothers themselves and of their husbands!

One may hesitate to tackle the measurement of indirect effects when the latter are numerous. Indeed, sometimes the chain of indirect effects may never end. The objection is understandable. In that case one needs a modeling approach to evaluation because the scheme of interactions becomes too complicated to be handled well by CBA.

3.6. STUDYING COST-BENEFIT ANALYSIS BY MEANS OF HYPOTHETICAL PROBLEMS[10]

We know from above that the fundamental choice rule is that a project whose net present value is positive can be adopted. In a number of cases variants of or deviations from this rule are appropriate, however. We will study the NPV rule and related choice rules in the following series of hypothetical problems:

3.6.1. DECIDING ON A SINGLE PROJECT

In a certain rural area, the project consists of providing primary health care by 5 health workers. The latter are recruited among the population. The cost of the project consists of the benefits foregone by shifting the workers from agricultural work to health services plus the cost of educating the health workers. There are three types of benefits from this primary health care project:

Type A: increase of agricultural production due to
a reduction in infant and child mortality
Type B: increase of agricultural production due to
a reduction in adult mortality
Type C: increase of agricultural production due to
a decrease in adult morbidity.

Assume that the cost-benefit analyst takes account of a period of 20 years; this implies that he
considers that there are no net benefits beyond a
20 year period. We will, furthermore, assume the
following: benefits due to lower morbidity amount
to 10,000 $ yearly, benefits due to the decrease in
adult mortality amount to 15,000 $ yearly whereas
benefits due to the decrease in infant and child
mortality amount to 30,000 $ yearly from the 15th
year to the 20th year[11]. The opportunity cost of
educating the health workers is 2,000 $ in the first
year only. The opportunity cost of the health care
work of the five health workers is put at 5,000 $
yearly. The social discount rate used is 10 per
cent. The exercise of calculating net present values is done in Table 3.1. It can be seen that the
net present value exceeds by far zero which means
that the project may certainly be adopted.

3.6.2. DECIDING BETWEEN ALTERNATIVE PROJECTS

Suppose a rural district's government has to make a
choice between a rural health center that emphasizes
immunization, a rural health center that provides
immunization and malaria control and a health center
that, apart from malaria control and immunization,
engages in nutrition education and administers nutrition supplements if needed. Let us call the three
alternatives projects I, II and III respectively.
The types of benefit are identical to those defined
in the previous exercise.

The opportunity costs of the three alternative
projects are assumed here to be equal to the expenditures made for each project (cost of building,
wages of personnel, cost of drugs, *etc.*). As before we will make the hypotheses that the cost-
benefit analyst performs his calculations over a
period of 20 years, that the benefits from reduced
infant and child mortality start in the 15th year
and that the social discount rate is 10 per cent.
In Table 3.2 a summary is given of costs and benefits. It can be seen that project II should be

Table 3.1. Deciding on a single project

Sources of costs	Present value of costs ($)	Sources of benefits	Present value of benefits ($)
1. Cost of education of health workers	2,000	1. Higher production due to reduction in child and infant mortality (Type A)	$30{,}000 \times \sum_{t=15}^{20} \frac{1}{1.10^{t-1}} = 37{,}846.8$
2. Opportunity cost of health care work	$5{,}000 \times \sum_{t=1}^{20} \frac{1}{1.10^{t-1}} = 46{,}824.6$	2. Higher production due to reduction of adult mortality (Type B)	$15{,}000 \times \sum_{t=1}^{20} \frac{1}{1.10^{t-1}} = 140{,}473.8$
		3. Higher production due to reduction of adult morbidity (Type C)	$10{,}000 \times \sum_{t=1}^{20} \frac{1}{1.10^{t-1}} = 93{,}649.2$
SUBTOTAL	48,824.6	SUBTOTAL	= 271,969.8

NET PRESENT VALUE = 223,145.2

Table 3.2. Deciding between alternative projects

Project	Type of benefit	Yearly benefits (฿)	Present value of benefits (฿)	Yearly costs (฿)	Present value of costs (฿)	Net present value (฿)
I	A	30,000	37,846.8			
	B	10,000	93,649.2			
	C	5,000	46,824.6			
			Total 178,320.6	10,000	Total 93,649.2	84,671.4
II	A	40,000	50,462.4			
	B	15,000	140,473.8			
	C	10,000	93,649.2			
			Total 284,585.4	15,000	Total 140,473.8	144,111.6
III	A	42,000	52,985.5			
	B	17,000	159,203.6			
	C	12,000	112,379.0			
			Total 324,568.1	20,000	Total 187,298.4	137,269.7

chosen since it entails the highest net present value.

3.6.3. DECIDING ON THE SCALE OF A PROJECT

In the example above, three alternative projects with different characteristics were studied. It is possible now that alternative projects have essentially the same characteristics but that they differ in size. The example we will treat is that of a rural health center that can employ five different quantities of health workers. We will consider the same types of benefits as above. The total cost has two components: first, there is the initial cost of educating the health workers and secondly, a yearly cost equal to the foregone benefits from not putting the health workers to work in agriculture. The period of all projects is 20 years while the social discount rate is again 10 per cent.

The cost-benefit analysis is summarized in Table 3.3. The result of the analysis is that the health center with 15 health workers is optimal. The analysis can also be depicted graphically in Figure 3.2. Although we have (imaginary) data for only 5 projects, it is possible to have an idea of the continuous distribution of benefits and costs if we link all points B and C on Figure 3.2. On the figure, it can be clearly seen that the highest net benefit is secured by the third project (with 15 health workers), since at that project's size marginal benefit of an additional health worker just equals the marginal cost of an extra health worker.

3.6.4. DECIDING ON A COMBINATION OF PROJECTS WHEN THERE IS A CONSTRAINT ON THEIR TOTAL FINANCIAL COST

Up to here we have treated problems for which financial constraints on projects were absent. Let us now study the example of a certain rural district that has only limited budgets available for health projects. It therefore has to choose an optimal combination of health projects. The list of possible projects is the following:
    I.   1 hospital
    II. 1 health center with 5 health workers
    III. sanitation education program

Table 3.3. Choosing the size of the health personnel in a rural health center

Size of project (in number of health workers)	Type of benefit	Yearly benefits (฿)	Present value of benefits (฿)	Yearly costs (฿)	Present value of costs (฿)	Net present value (฿)
5	A	30,000	37,846.8		2,000.0	
	B	15,000	140,473.8		46,824.6	
	C	10,000	93,649.2	5,000		
	Total		271,969.8		48,824.6	223,145.2
10	A	35,000	44,154.6		4,000.0	
	B	18,000	168,568.6		93,649.2	
	C	14,000	131,108.9	10,000		
	Total		343,832.1		97,649.2	246,182.9
15	A	38,000	47,939.3		6,000.0	
	B	20,500	191,980.9		140,473.8	
	C	16,500	154,521.2	15,000		
	Total		394,441.4		146,473.8	247,967.6
20	A	40,000	50,462.4		8,000.0	
	B	21,000	196,663.3		187,298.4	
	C	18,000	168,568.6	20,000		
	Total		415,694.3		195,298.4	220,395.9
25	A	41,000	51,724.0		10,000.0	
	B	21,500	201,345.8		234,123.0	
	C	19,000	177,933.5	25,000		
	Total		431,003.3		244,123,0	186,880.3

Figure 3.2. Costs and benefits of rural health
centers of different sizes, in thousand
$

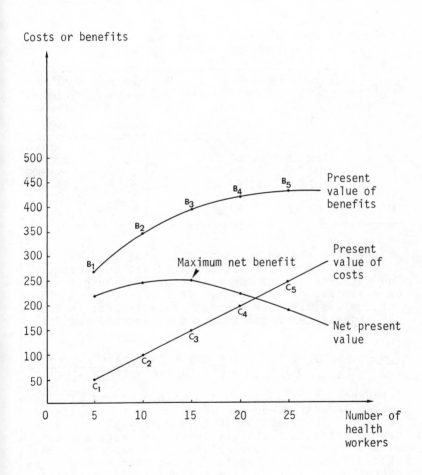

V. nutrition supplements program
VI. birth control program

For each project one calculates as before its net present value (NPV) and the *NPV-financial cost ratio*. Subsequently one ranks the projects according to this ratio. One accepts the projects starting from the top of the ranking until one has exhausted the present value of the budget. We will illustrate this procedure in Table 3.4, omitting this time the explicit calculation of costs and benefits.

Table 3.4. Optimal combination of projects given a budget constraint

Project	Net present value (ℬ)	Present value of financial costs (ℬ)	NPV-financial cost-ratio	Cumulative financial costs (ℬ)
I	1,750,000	700,000	2.5	700,000
II	175,000	100,000	1.75	800,000
V	80,000	50,000	1.6	850,000
III	120,000	80,000	1.5	930,000
VI	130,000	100,000	1.3	1,030,000
IV	60,000	50,000	1.2	1,080,000

If the budget is limited to 850,000 ℬ, it follows that projects I, II and V are to be chosen. The net benefits of the health project budget will be maximized in that case. This procedure is indeed very plausible: one chooses those project that have the highest net benefits per discounted ℬ spent.

3.6.5. DECIDING ON ALLOCATING A CONSTRAINED RESOURCE IN A PROJECT SUBJECT TO A BUDGET CONSTRAINT

Frequently one is confronted with problems of allocating inputs between *subprograms* of a health project. The question in that case will be how one has to allocate available inputs in order to maximize a project's net benefits. The example we will study is that of a health project that involves the operation of a hospital and a rural health center. Let us suppose at the outset that there is only one medical doctor available and that he will be allocated to the hospital. Given a fixed budget, only

10 health workers can be recruited: these are to be allocated between the hospital and the rural health center. The allocation rule is that the allocation of health workers is optimal only if the marginal net benefits of working in the hospital (MB_h) and the marginal net benefits of working in the rural health center (MB_r) are equalized. Indeed, as long as MB_r exceeds MB_g, it pays to shift a health worker from the hospital to the rural center.

In Table 3.5, a list is given of the marginal net benefits of the health workers. One can imagine that these benefits are composed of the same types of benefits as in 3.6.1. The procedure one has to follow is to see where each succeeding health worker has the highest value. The decision by which 6 workers will be allocated to the rural center and 4 workers to the hospital is optimal, since at that allocation marginal net benefits are equalized. It is an optimal combination because total net benefits can no longer be improved.

Table 3.5. Marginal net benefits of health workers in a rural health center and a hospital

Health worker number	Rural health center	Health worker number	Hospital
1	51,000	1	48,400
2	50,000	2	48,300
3	49,500	3	48,200
4	49,000	4 (*)	48,000
5	48,500	5	47,900
6 (*)	48,000	6	47,800
7	47,500	7	47,700
8	47,500	8	47,600
9	46,500	9	47,500
10	46,000	10	47,400

(*) refers to the optimal solution.

3.6.6. DECIDING ON THE ALLOCATION OF VARIOUS RESOURCES IN A SINGLE PROJECT SUBJECT TO A BUDGET CONSTRAINT

Here we will study how various resources have to be allocated in a primary health care project. The project has benefits in $ (B) that are related to the various project inputs. As inputs, we define physicians' time (r_1), midwives' and nurses' time (r_2), health workers' time (r_3) and drugs (r_4); time of health personnel is expressed in hours. The benefit function can be written as

$$B = B(r_1, r_2, r_3, r_4) \qquad (3.3)$$

The budget constraint faced by the project manager is

$$p_1 r_1 + p_2 r_2 + p_3 r_3 + p_4 r_4 = R \qquad (3.4)$$

where R refers to the budget in $, p_1, p_2 and p_3 to the hourly wage rate of physicians, nurses and health workers, respectively, and p_4 to the (uniform) price of drugs.

The project manager can now maximize (3.3) (subject to (3.4)) by differentiating the Lagrangean function[12] with respect to the inputs and setting results equal to zero. The Lagrangean function to be maximized is

$$\text{Max } B(r_1, r_2, r_3, r_4) - \lambda\{p_1 r_1 + p_2 r_2 + p_3 r_3 + p_4 r_4 - R\}$$

The optimal choice of the four resources can be obtained from the following first order conditions

$$\frac{\partial B}{\partial r_1} - \lambda p_1 = 0$$

$$\frac{\partial B}{\partial r_2} - \lambda p_2 = 0$$

$$\frac{\partial B}{\partial r_3} - \lambda p_3 = 0$$

$$\frac{\partial B}{\partial r_4} - \lambda p_4 = 0$$

$$p_1 r_1 + p_2 r_2 + p_3 r_3 + p_4 r_4 - R = 0$$

The first four order conditions can be rewritten as:

$$\frac{\dfrac{\partial B}{\partial r_i}}{\dfrac{\partial B}{\partial r_j}} = \frac{p_i}{p_j} \qquad \begin{array}{l} \text{for all i and j} \\ \text{and } i \neq j \end{array} \qquad (3.5)$$

where $i=1,2,3,4$ and $j=1,2,3,4$. The left-hand side of (3.5) represents the *marginal rate of substitution* (MRS) in the benefit between inputs i and j. In other words it represents the amount of input i that is needed as a substitute for j in order for the benefit to remain constant; it is assumed thereby that the amount of inputs other than i and j cannot be changed.

Let us now for a moment make abstraction of inputs r_3 and r_4 and assume that the problem at hand is one of allocating physicians'time and nurses'time in an optimal manner. By totally differentiating B and setting the result equal to 0, one has

$$dB = \frac{\partial B}{\partial r_1} dr_1 + \frac{\partial B}{\partial r_2} dr_2 = 0$$

so that
$$\frac{\frac{\partial B}{\partial r_1}}{\frac{\partial B}{\partial r_2}} = - \frac{dr_2}{dr_1}$$

As long as(3.5) does not hold for $i=1$ and $j=2$, one can improve the objective. Indeed, one can for instance state that when $-dr_2/dr_1$ is smaller than p_1/p_2, it pays to increase the use of nurses'time and decreases the use of physicians' time. Suppose that $-dr_2/dr_1$ has the hypothetical value of 2 and that p_1/p_2 is 4. The latter price ratio means that one can receive in the market 4 hours of nurses'time by giving up 1 hours of physician's time. However the MRS indicates that it only takes two hours of nurses'time as a substitute for one hour of physicians'time to keep the same benefit. By performing an exchange between r_1 and r_2 in the market,one can therefore make total benefit rise!

It is easy to depict the numerical example given in Figure 3.3. The straight line in Figure 3.3 represents the budget line; the absolute value of its slope is 4. The curves are *benefit isoquants*, *i.e.* lines that represent all possible combinations of nurses' and physicians' time that will guarantee a certain benefit level. The higher the isoquant is located in the graph, the higher the level of B. At point B_1, it can be seen that the MRS ($-dr_2/dr_1$) is smaller than the absolute value of the scope of the budget line (p_1/p_2). Moving away from B_1, thereby using more nurses'time and less physicians'time, is a move towards the optimum. The substitution of

Figure 3.3. Optimal allocation of nurses' and
physicians' time in a health care
project

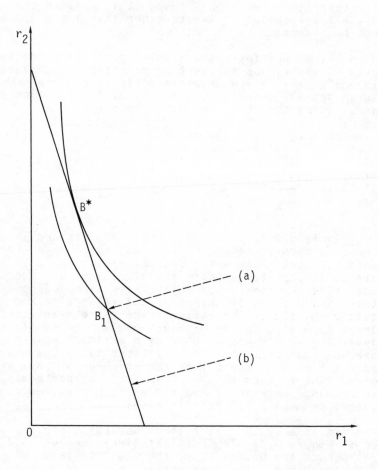

Notes: (a) : at B_1, absolute value of the slope of the

isoquant $= -\dfrac{dr_2}{dr_1} = 2$

(b) : at any point on the budget line, absolute

value of the slope of the budget line $= \dfrac{p_1}{p_2} = 4$

r_1 by r_2 has to be continued until the point $B^{\ddagger}$ is reached; that point represents an optimum since further improvements of the objective B are impossible.

3.6.7. DISTRIBUTIONAL CONSIDERATIONS IN THE COST-BENEFIT ANALYSIS OF A PROJECT

It is sometimes said that issues of income distribution are to be kept out of CBA. However, in many circumstances, it is hard to circumvent the distribution problem. To illustrate this, suppose that in a certain city, the city government has the choice between building an extra hospital and setting up additional primary health care (PHC) centers in the city. In the hospital only curative services will be provided, whereas the PHC centers deliver preventive as well as curative services. Let us assume that the PHC centers deliver free services whereas the hospital charges fees. Additional (progressive) taxes are supposed to make the city budget balance.

One can imagine that the PHC centers are more directly accessible to the city's poor. Compared to the hospital, the centers are likely to contribute much more to the poor's well-being since they provide preventive services such as sanitation and nutrition education and family planning instruction. In Table 3.6, the net benefits of the two alternative projects for the different income categories are compared. Net benefits are measured in terms of net income gained[13] as a result of the health projects.

Table 3.6. Net benefits of two alternative health
          interventions in a city

Income category	Hospital	PHC centers
Upper income population group	300	-50
Middle income population group	400	100
Poor population group	100	650
City's total population	800	700

In the example, the hospital project results in higher benefits for the upper and middle income group than for the poor. One can indeed imagine that people in the former groups make a greater use of the hospital services because they can more easily afford to pay the hospital fees. Since earnings are used to calculate the monetary equivalent of higher productivity, less mortality and morbidity, the first two groups' benefits are higher than the benefits to the poor. Notice that the poor are the major beneficiaries of the PHC intervention. The reason is that the various PHC services will render the poor much healthier. As a result their labor participation can be increased which in turn leads to a better income status.

According to previous choice rules, the hospital should be preferred to the PHC centers because total net benefits of the hospital (800) exceed those of the PHC centers (700). The city government can reason that on equity grounds, the PHC project should be preferred because the poor are much better off than in the hospital project. This would mean that *implicitly* a high *distribution weight* is given to the gains of the poor. In other words, the city would attribute a higher social marginal utility of income to the poor than to the richer categories. It also signifies that the city government judges that the distributional gains offset the loss in efficiency, measured here by the loss of society's income. Note that the latter amounts to 100.

It is also feasible to assign explicit weights, on an *ex-ante* basis, to the net gains of the various population groups. A possibility, already mentioned before, would be to use as weight, the average national income divided by the average income of the population group considered; the latter would mean that the weights decrease as the population groups become richer.

3.7. CASE STUDY I: ECONOMIC ASPECTS OF ASCARIS INFECTION IN KENYA

3.7.1. INTRODUCTION

This is a study undertaken by Latham *et al*. (1977) of the World Bank in order, firstly, to estimate how much ascariasis (infection by roundworms) is costing to Kenyans in terms of health care costs and in

terms of costs to private citizens and, secondly,
to estimate the costs of feasible programs to control ascaris infection[14]. The analysis is done for
the year 1976.

Note that ascariasis entails a malabsorption
of various nutrients. The authors' research had
indicated, for instance, that heavy infections can
lead to non-utilization of 25 per cent of ingested
calories. In the next section, we will give an
overview of the current costs associated with ascariasis. In section 3.7.3, an alternative way to
control ascariasis will be described. If the latter
is implemented, it follows that the current costs
(see 3.7.2) will be saved; these are regarded as an
estimate of the benefits of the alternative ascariasis control program. These cost savings will be
compared with the costs of the alternative control
program. The resulting net cost savings are interpreted as the net benefits to Kenyan society.

3.7.2. CURRENT COSTS OF ASCARIASIS

Health care cost
Using a prevalence rate of 25 per cent, the
estimated number of ascariasis infected persons in
Kenya is 3,474,000 in 1976. It was further estimated that only 2.6 per cent of those persons were
treated at government hospitals, either as inpatients
or outpatients. The number of inpatients and outpatients is 1,324 and 87,480 respectively. Since
government hospitals amount to around half of the
country's hospitals, the figures above have been
doubled to get an estimate of Kenya's hospital
ascariasis-patients. The cost per outpatient (ex-
cluding medication) is estimated at 0.5 $ whereas
the cost per inpatient is 35 $ for a 7-day stay at
the hospital. Total costs are estimated to be $
180,160. Note that the latter underestimates the
real cost, since outpatients treated at rural health
centers or dispensaries are not included in the
analysis (due to a lack of data).

Cost of anthelmintics
The total cost of anthelmintics was estimated
to be 159,462 $ in 1976. This figure is based upon
purchases by Central Medical Stores (that supply
government and mission hospitals outside Nairobi)
and purchases by the Hospital Pharmacy at Nairobi's
Kenyatta National Hospital. In the final cost fig-

ure an estimate was included for the cost of anthelmintics used by private practitioners and hospitals not supplied by Central Medical Stores.

Cost of private citizens

The costs to families include the purchase of anthelmintics in retail stores, work-time lost and travel expenses for trips to hospitals and the food that is unabsorbed by infected persons due to the ascaris infection.

(i) Retail purchase of anthelmintics

It is assumed that 15 per cent of preschool children, 10 per cent of school-aged children and 5 per cent of adults purchase 1 dose or tablet of an anti-ascaris anthelmintic each year. The authors assumed further that the dose increases with age, namely a preschool child receives one tablet, a schoolchild receives 2 tablets and an adult receives 3 tablets. These assumptions mean that 15 per cent of the total Kenyan population receives 1 tablet per year. With a retail price per tablet of $ 0.094, private purchases amount to $ 195,469 (given a population of 13,900,000 in 1976).

(ii) Work-time lost and travel expenses

The authors assume that outpatients loose half a day's work by travelling to and from the hospital. Note that even if the outpatient is a child, an adult has to accompany the child resulting in loss of time. It is assumed that for inpatients, half of the patients are adults: these loose 7 days of work. The value of the loss of work is estimated at 0.875 $ per day (which has to be regarded as a minimum value since it is the wage applied to unskilled laborers). The value of transport to and from the hospital is estimated at 0.35 $ and 1.09 $ for the outpatients and inpatients respectively. It can then be calculated that the total amount of work-time lost and travel expenses is $ 199.168.

(iii) Food unabsorbed

Ascariasis is associated with decreased absorption of protein, fat and carbohydrate. This means that a certain amount of food is wasted due to the roundworms. The latter is of special importance given the already existing problem of malnutrition in Kenya.

Previous research by Tripathy *et.al.* (1971, 1972) on Colombian children has led to the conclusion that in children with a load of 66 worms, 26 per cent of total calories are lost due to worm infection[15] (5 per cent of calories lost as fat and 21 per cent lost as carbohydrate). It is further assumed that in Kenya, the average infected person has 7 worms. Assuming then that the loss of calories is proportional to the amount of worms, 7 worms lead to a loss of calories of 2.8 per cent. Given a theoretical daily average intake of 2,400 calories, the total daily loss of calories amounts to 233,520,000 (= 3,475,000 infected persons x 2,400 calories x 2.8 per cent). Kenyans receive 75 per cent of their food from maizemeal and 25 per cent from beans, milk, meat and vegetables. The latter food costs 0.30 $ per kg; it costs twice as much per kg as maizemeal. It is further supposed that the same amount of calories is derived from a kg of maize or non-maize food, namely 3,620. This means then that per year 23,545,420 kg of food is unabsorbed (= 233,520,000 calories x 365 days: 3,620 calories per kg). The value of this amount of food, taking account of the different costs for maize and non-maize food, amounts to 4,414,766 $ or 1.27 $ per infected Kenyan.

3.7.3. AN ALTERNATIVE CONTROL PROGRAM

Ascariasis is a disease which can be passed from person to person. Indeed, faeces of infected persons contain the worms' eggs. If someone gets somehow infective eggs on his fingers, he may be infected with ascaris after bringing them into contact with his mouth. It is evident that many children get the disease in this way. But adults are also prone to the disease. The disease could be eradicated when a substantial effort is undertaken in improving health education (children and adults can be educated how to prevent the transmission of the disease), and housing and sanitation (toilet construction is a way to stop bodily contact with infected faeces). Such improvements are not likely to occur very fast, however. Therefore, the authors reason that mass treatment of ascariasis by drugs is a recommendable control program. The drug treatment will bring about an important decrease of the likelihood that faeces contain the worms' eggs. As a result, transmission of the disease will also diminish substantially.

The authors mention that mass drug treatment of vulnerable groups has main medical and economic advantages over other control methods, namely
(i) the time and cost of stool examinations are saved;
(ii) it is a cost-effective method because for the same amount of money, many more persons can be treated than in conventional health care facilities;
(iii) the person that administers the drugs does not need a genuine medical training;
(iv) prevention and cure are combined in one delivery system.

The *costs of mass drug treatment* can be estimated after making the following assumptions:
(i) the type of drug chosen is levamisole that is a broad-spectrum drug; it is also active against other helminths like hookworm and trichuris. Its price is 0.035 $ per tablet;
(ii) from Kenya's population of 13,900,000 three age groups are derived: 14 per cent are in the group 1-4 years of age, 29 per cent in the group 5-14 years of age and 52 per cent in the group 16 years of age and over. The first group receives 1 tablet twice a year, the second group receives 2 tablets once a year and the third group receives 3 tablets once every 2 years. Note that children younger than 1 year are not treated.

Using these assumptions, the total cost amounts to 797,860 $.

3.7.4. SUMMARY OF COSTS AND BENEFITS OF DRUG TREATMENT

The summary is presented in Table 3.7. Let us emphasize that the benefits are put equal to the gross cost savings resulting from the implementation of the drug treatment program. It can be seen that the net cost savings due to this program amount to 4,351,165 $. At the same time this amount is an approximation of the net value of the drug treatment program. It follows that the alternative program will augment the Kenyans'welfare.

Table 3.7. Benefits and costs of ascariasis drug
         treatment program, in $ (1976)

Gross Cost Savings = Benefits		Costs of Drug Treatment	
1.Health care system (hospital treatment)		1.Drug treatment costs per age group	
1.1. Patient care	180,160	1 - 4 years old	136,220
1.2. Drugs	159,462	5 - 14 years old	282,170
subtotal	339,622	15 years and older	379,470
2.Family expenditure			
2.1. Retail purchase of drugs	195,469		
2.2. Lost wages, transport	199,168		
2.3. Food lost	4,414,766		
subtotal	4,809,403		
Total Benefits	5,149,025	Total Costs	797,860
Net Cost Savings = Net Value			4,351,165

3.7.5. CRICITAL COMMENTS

It has to be admitted that the savings of costs due
to mass drug treatment are substantial. The authors
themselves warn, however, that the benefits may
still be underestimated. Indeed, the benefits do
not include the cost savings of treating patients
in rural health centers or dispensaries. The calculated benefits also exclude the benefits associated
with the control of hookworm, trichuris and
strongyloides infections made possible by the broad
spectrum drug. Note that it has been estimated by
Basta and Churchill (1974) that heavy hookworm infection leads to a productivity decrease of unskilled workers by 15 to 20 per cent. Eradication of
hookworms is therefore likely to entail supplemen-
tary productivity benefits. Unfortunately, the
study fails to measure these. Furthermore, on the
cost side of the cost-benefit analysis, the cost of
the delivery system of the drugs has been omitted.

Further points of critique can be raised. *First,*
the cost-benefit analysis is static. The costs savings due to application to the drug treatment program are likely to be repeated yearly. Hence, it is

preferable to make an estimate of net cost savings in the future and to calculate subsequently the net present value of benefits. *Secondly*, it is doubtful whether the drug treatment will be 100 per cent effective at once. Indeed, the delivery system may not be functioning adequately or groups of people may fail to take the drug. Moreover, new infections caused by unhygienic habits may occur. Thus, it would be recommendable to make an estimate of the costs of prolonged necessary drug treatment. *Thirdly*, in order to measure the value of work-time lost, the authors use a 'representative wage for unskilled work in Kenya'[16]. It is not clear to us whether this wage corresponds to marginal productivity. If this representative wage exceeds marginal productivity, the amount corresponding to item 2.2 in Table 3.7 will be overestimated. A similar problem is that of the price of drugs. The drugs have to be imported and have to be paid in hard currency. It should certainly be checked whether the official exchange rate corresponds to the true willingness to pay for a unit of hard currency. If the latter is not the case, the shadow price of foreign exchange should be used in calculating the local price of imported drugs. It is clear that the drug treatment costs will be underestimated if the shadow price of foreign exchange exceeds the official exchange rate. *Fourthly*, it is well known that fecally related diseases such as ascariasis could be eradicated if the sanitary environment were excellent. Such a condition can only be the result of continued health education (leading to appropriate use of toilets, the use of clean water, washing hands before eating *etc.*) and of investments in sanitation (toilet construction, provision of clear water *etc.*). The authors say that a healthy environment will only be attained in the long run, hence it is not a real alternative to drug treatment. Nevertheless, it would be useful to do the cost-benefit analysis of an intervention in the sanitary environment as well. Indeed, the fact that such an intervention produces only benefits in the long run does not have to lead to an automatic rejection. It is only by comparing the net present values of alternatives that we can judge what is best for society. *Fifthly*, we remind the reader that the benefits that result from applying the cost-savings approach to benefit calculation are to be seen as an approximation of the true welfare benefits that follow from a WTP approach.

3.8. CASE STUDY II: THE ECONOMIC COSTS AND BENEFITS OF AN IMMUNIZATION PROGRAM IN INDONESIA

3.8.1. INTRODUCTION

The study presented below is that of Barnum (1981). It applies CBA to an expanded immunization program in Indonesia. The program consists of the delivery of BCG (tuberculosis) and DPT (diphteria, pertussis and tetanus) vaccinations in two visits during the first year of life, and TFT (tetanus) vaccinations of pregnant women. BCG vaccinations are also to be given to children entering and leaving school.

This immunization program is planned over a five-year period, beginning with the fiscal year 1979-1980. Its main objective is to reduce infant and child morbidity and mortality. CBA is carried out for four types of interventions: the total program, DPT (henceforth including TFT) only, BCG only as well as BCG marginal to the DPT program. The costs of a program are put equal to that program's financial cost. The benefits consist of *cost savings* (avoided treatment costs plus the avoided cost of time spent by mothers in home care) and *income* gained as a result of prevented mortality.

3.8.2. PREVENTION OF CASES AND DEATHS BY THE PROGRAM

First, one calculates, on the basis of disease attack rates and case fatality rates, how many children would attract the disease and die in the absence of intervention. *Secondly,* one calculates each program's effectiveness. The latter is equal to the vaccine efficacy times the program coverage in terms of population. Subsequently, it can be derived how many cases and deaths will be averted thanks to the immunization interventions.

Note that in the case of DPT, one takes account only of the number of cases and deaths prevented during the first five years of life. In the case of BCG for infants, the cases and deaths prevented during the first ten years of life are considered; concerning BCG vaccinations for the children entering school (at age six to seven), a ten year period is selected as well. The prevented cases and deaths due to BCG vaccinations of children leaving school are omitted from the analysis. In Table 3.8 information is given on the potential action of the im-

83

munization programs.

Table 3.8. Potential number of cases and deaths
            prevented by the immunization program

Year	DPT & TFT		BCG		Total	
	Cases	Deaths	Cases	Deaths	Cases	Deaths
1979-80	119,640	14,446	1,670	276	121,310	14,822
1980-81	252,682	23,012	3,439	773	256,121	23,785
1981-82	421,161	36,736	5,358	1,205	426,519	37,942
1982-83	596,744	47,439	7,442	1,675	604,186	49,114
1983-84	774,107	57,756	9,549	2,150	783,656	59,906
1984-85	506,235	16,449	11,368	2,556	517,603	19,005
1985-86	319,990	11,428	13,742	3,093	333,742	14,521
1986-87	222,622	7,110	16.371	3,682	238,993	10,792
1987-88	119,367	3,980	19,269	4,336	138,636	8,316
1988-89			22,312	5,019	22,312	5,019
1989-90			18,896	4,252	18,896	4,252
1990-91			14,688	3,305	14,688	3,305
1991-92			10,102	2,272	10,102	2,272
1992-93			5,109	1,149	5,109	1,149
Total	3,332,908	218,356	159,315	35,844	3,492,223	254,200

Source: Barnum (1981, p.5).

3.8.3. PROGRAM COSTS

The costs consist of the project expenditures minus
the value of the capital that is left at the end of
the fifth year of the project. Special attention
has to be paid to the cost calculation of the programs separately. The total value of the capital
expenditures for cold chain and transportation has
to be included in both the cost of DPT and BCG.
However, expenditures for vaccines, vaccine production development, syringes *etc.* can be allocated in
an appropriate way to the separate programs. The
program costs for the alternative interventions are
given in Table 3.9.

3.8.4. PROGRAM BENEFITS

Avoided treatment costs
      First, we have the costs of treatment by tra-
ditional means (jamu medicine): these costs are un-

necessary if the diseases considered are absent.
One reckons that approximately 75 per cent of the
sick would make use of traditional medecine. The
expenditures per symptom week for DPT (two weeks)
and tuberculosis (thirty weeks) amount to 75 and 50
Rupiah (Rp.), respectively. This implies that total
costs of traditional medecine avoided are equal to
112.5 (=.75 x 75 Rp. x 2) times the number of DPT
cases prevented plus 1125 (=.75 x 50 Rp. x 30)times
the number of tuberculosis cases prevented.

Secondly, there are the costs of modern medical
care that are not needed in the event of immunization.
It is estimated that 7 per cent of households use
modern medical care. The total of avoided treatment
costs are obtained by multiplying 7 per cent times
the cost of treatment times the number of cases prevented. Note that inpatient care is required for
treatment of tetanus and diphteria whereas outpatient care is usual for tuberculosis and pertussis.
The cost estimates are 45000 Rp. per case of diphteria, 6000 Rp. per case of pertussis, 55000 Rp.
per case of tetanus and 49000 Rp. per case of tuberculosis.

Value of mothers' time spent in home care
The value of mothers' care avoided represents a
welfare gain: indeed, mothers can put in more agricultural work if their children remain unharmed as
a result of the immunization program. The shadow
wage of mothers is based now upon the results of a
labor participation survey: it is equal to one-half
of the average wage during the busy agricultural
season whereas it is one-fourth of the average wage
during the slack season. Note that the busy season
is about one-fourth of the calendar year. The value
of mothers' time over the calendar year is then
equal to

$$w(\frac{1}{4} \cdot \frac{1}{2} + \frac{3}{4} \cdot \frac{1}{4}) \cdot d \cdot c$$

where w is the average wage rate, d is the number
of days lost for production per illness and c represents the number of prevented cases. It is further assumed that d is seven for tuberculosis and 3
for DPT.

Income gains from prevented mortality
It is assumed that the child which is saved
from disease enters the labor market at age twelve.
He receives a starting wage of one-fourth the na-

Table 3.9. Cost-benefit analysis of Indonesian immunization program (Rp. × 10⁶)

Year	Total immunization program (DPT-TFT & BCG)		DPT-TFT Program only		BCG Program only		BCG as an added program	
	Costs	Benefits[1]	Costs[2]	Benefits[1]	Costs[2]	Benefits[1]	Costs[3]	Benefits[1]
1979-80	2541	1400	2268	1328	1388	72	273	72
1980-81	2654	2486	2384	2319	1457	167	270	167
1981-82	2943	4228	2641	3936	1531	291	302	291
1982-83	3379	6378	3052	5927	1785	450	327	450
1983-84	3623	7795	3267	7148	1817	646	356	646
1984-85	-1332[4]	3716	-1311[4]	2649	-1217[4]	1067	-21[4]	1067
1985-86		4183		2555		1628		1628
1986-87		4092		1836		2256		2256
1987-88		4098		1144		2954		2954
1988-89		3104				3104		3104
1989-90		3305				3305		3305
1990-91		2667				2667		2667
1991-92		1901				1901		1901
1992-93		997				997		997
Net present value at 15 %		12196		7156		1322		5040

[1]This is the undiscounted value of total benefits accruing to the program in the column heading.
[2]This represents the cost of operating a BCG program without a DPT program (or conversely for column three). The costs of operating the two programs separately do not add up to the costs of the total program since much of the total costs are for shared expenditures.
[3]This represents the added cost if a BCG program is considered additional to a DPT program.
[4]Value of capital remaining at the end of five years.

Source: Barnum (1981, p.12).

tional average income. His wage then increases
gradually up to the national average at age 20.
From the age of 20 to 55, his income continues to
increase at an average of 4 per cent per year.
Using a discount rate of 15 per cent and taking account of survival probabilities, one can calculate
for each group and for each year of the analysis
the present value of lifetime earnings. The latter
constitute a gain since they would not have been
realized in the absence of immunization programs.

3.8.5. SUMMARY OF THE COST-BENEFIT ANALYSIS

In Table 3.9 four cost-benefit analyses are presented. Remember that the costs are equal to the program's financial cost whereas the benefits are the
sum of avoided treatment costs, the value of mothers'time spent in home care and the income generated
as a result of prevented mortality.

It is clear that the total immunization
program is economically viable, its net present value (given a discount rate of 15 per cent) being
12196 (10^6)Rp. The program consisting only of DPT and
TFT immunizations would also represent a new welfare
gain to Indonesian society. The BCG program, when
operated as a separate program, has a fairly low
net present value compared to the two previously
cited programs. Barnum (1981, p.13) also states
that this particular result does not withstand a
sensitivity test. For instance, with an increase
in costs of 25 per cent and a decrease in benefits
of 33 per cent, net present value becomes negative.
Hence, running the BCG program separately does not
seem to represent a welfare gain. However, when
the BCG program is added to the DPT-TFT program, a
satisfactory result is obtained. In other words,
'it is found that a program which is not economically viable by itself becomes viable when added as
one component of a larger immunization program'[17].

It follows that a similar result would probably
be obtained if we would investigate the costs and
benefits of the addition of other immunization programs,such as polio and measles.

3.8.6. CRITICAL COMMENTS

A number of shortcomings are admitted by the author

himself. The estimates are likely to be conserva-
tive because, first, only the direct effects of immunization are included; in other words, the beneficial effects of reduced transmission of the diseases
is not taken account of. Secondly, the effect of
BCG immunization of children completing school is
not measured. Thirdly, the effect of TFT on maternal
morbidity and mortality is omitted from the analysis.

Some additional remarks concern the program
costs. One may wonder to what extent the various
types of equipment have to be imported. It is evident that, if imports occur, it needs to be checked
whether the foreign exchange rate reflects the true
willingness to pay of the Indonesian consumer. One
also notices that the value of capital remaining at
the end of the project is deducted from program
costs. This implies that it is considered to be a
benefit. The latter is only correct, however, if
the remaining capital can be used fully again in
the economy at large. If this proves to be a false
hypothesis, the remaining capital needs to be clas-
sified as a cost, of course. Concerning the benefit
calculation, Barnum has used cost savings and income
gained as measures of benefit. We remind the reader
once again that they only constitute an approximation of the true benefits measured by society's
willingness to pay for the programs.

NOTES
    [1] Stated more precisely, marginal utility of
medical care is equal to AB up to a certain constant;
this constant is equal to the marginal utility of
income.
    [2] Strictly speaking this is only true if the
individual's real income is kept constant as one
moves along the demand curve. In that case the
latter is called a compensated demand curve.
    [3] See especially Broome (1978) on this point.
Note that health interventions may involve a reduction in the *risk* of death. In those cases the WTP
may be expected to be finite,however; see Mooney
et al. (1980, p.51).
    [4] The distinction between mortality, morbidity
and debility is taken from Mushkin (1962).
    [5] See UNIDO (1972, ch.5) on this issue.
    [6] At each quantity of labor, the corresponding
point on the demand for labor curve reflects the
value of marginal productivity.
    [7] See UNIDO (1972, ch.13).

[8] See also Dasgupta and Pierce (1978, ch.6).

[9] *Ibidem* (pp.61-69).

[10] This way of studying CBA is inspired by Stokey & Zeckhauser (1978).

[11] This is the result of an assumption that the first cohort of children saved during the first year of the project join the labor force at the age of 15.

[12] On Lagrangean functions, see *e.g.* Chiang (1967, pp.350-354).

[13] Net income can be gained as a result of higher productivity, less mortality and morbidity *etc.*; average earnings per category can be used to calculate the benefit in monetary terms.

[14] A published paper based on Latham *et al.* (1977) is Stephenson *et al.* (1980).

[15] The calculation does not take account of protein losses.

[16] See Stephenson *et al.* (1980, p.255).

[17] Barnum (1981, p.13).

Chapter Four

COST-EFFECTIVENESS ANALYSIS

4.1. DEFINITION

Cost-effectiveness analysis (CEA) is a method that
enables the health researcher to determine the
cheapest technique or system to meet a well defined
quantified target, or to determine the optimal
technique or system in order to maximize (or minimize) a particular non-quantified objective given
a fixed budget. An example of a problem that can
be analyzed using CEA is the following. Suppose
that the target of a health project in a certain
country is to reduce the infant mortality rate from
139 per thousand to 60 per thousand children within
5 years. CEA has to find out which type of health
intervention can guarantee that this target is met
at least financial cost. Alternatively, the health
project may be given a certain budget and may have
the objective of minimizing infant mortality. In
that case one searches for a health intervention
method that precisely minimizes the infant mortality while respecting the financial constraint.

It is clear that CEA is very different from
CBA. A first difference is that the target or objective is already given in CEA. In other words,
one does not have to occupy oneself with the question whether there are possibly other targets or
objectives with a higher social value. In this way,
CEA is easier to use because one does not have to
be concerned with the social or ethical values of
alternatives. This does not imply, however, that
CEA is free from value judgments. Indeed, any target or objective is loaded, implicitly, with value
judgments. The second difference is that targets
or objectives do not necessarily have to be measured
in money as in CBA; frequently they are expressed

90

in terms of health status indicators.

4.2. ELEMENTS OF COST-EFFECTIVENESS ANALYSIS

4.2.1. OPTIMAL CHOICE GIVEN A CERTAIN BUDGET

Choosing among alternatives

We begin by studying the hypothetical example of organizing a child health care system in a rural area. We will suppose that the objective is to maximize the decrease in infant mortality given a budget ot 100,000 $. Three *alternatives that exactly satisfy the budget constraint* are available: the operation of two stationary child health centers in the area (10 primary health care workers are attached to each center), the operation of one stationary child health center in a centrally located village (30 primary health care workers are attached to this center), and the operation of a mobile health unit that serves every village in the area twice a month. The three alternatives with their expected impact on infant mortality are listed in Table 4.1.

Table 4.1. Alternative child health care systems (with identical cost)

Alternative		Decrease in infant mortality (in ‰)
I	two stationary child health centers	40
II	one stationary child health center	30
III	mobile health unit	50

Is is easy to calculate the *impact ratio* for each alternative: it is the ratio of the decrease in infant mortality to the financial cost. These ratios are 0.0004, 0.0003 and 0.0005 for alternatives I, II and III, respectively; they are also called *figures of merit* by Seiler (1969, p.74). The choice to be made is fairly simple, *viz.* one selects the alternative with the highest impact ratio. It follows that alternative III is the most cost-effective choice since per dollar spent this alternative has the largest impact on infant mortality.

Very often the choice problem is not that simple. Frequently one has to choose between *alternatives having different health outcomes as well as different financial costs*. This problem will be studied by means of a second example. Suppose again that, in a rural area, the objective is to minimize infant mortality by setting up an optimal child health care system. Imagine the six hypothetical alternatives listed in Table 4.2. If the budget is limited to 1500,000 $, for instance, only projects I to IV are to be compared. However, it no longer follows that the alternative with the highest impact ratio is to be chosen. Indeed, if the third alternative (with an impact ratio of 0.0417) would be selected, we would not minimize infant mortality! Instead, as can be verified, alternative IV should be our best choice: it guarantees the lowest infant mortality while respecting the budget constraint. Notice that it is not compulsory for the most cost-effective option to exhaust the budget. One also sees in Table 4.2 that the mortality rate can be decreased still further if only the budget were larger. Here, we arrive into the realm of CBA. Decision-makers would have to decide whether a further decrease in infant mortality of 10 per thousand (made possible by project VI) is worth giving up an additional 300,000 $. The latter is clearly an issue that cannot be solved by CEA.

Choosing a combination of interventions
In a number of cases, the problem is not to choose between alternatives but to select an optimal combination of interventions. Imagine an anti-parasitic campaign in a rural district with the primary aim to reduce morbidity among adult males. The choice of this aim by the rural district's government is logical if it wants to reduce the loss of production due to the parasitic diseases. In Table 4.3, we list of a number of anti-parasitic eradication programs together with their (hypothetical) costs and impact on morbidity. Suppose that this rural district can count on a budget of 2000,000 $. The way to proceed is to rank the programs according to their impact ratios. One then selects the programs starting from the top of the list until the budget is exhausted. One can see from Table 4.4 that the programs against hookworm, malaria and schistosomiasis constitute the optimal combination.

Table 4.2. Alternative child health care systems
(with different financial cost)

Child health care system	Financial cost (in 1000$) (1)	Decrease in infant mortality (in ‰) (2)	Impact ratio (3)=(2)/(1)
I Health center (curative services only)	1000	30.0	.0300
II Health center I plus immunization	1150	40.0	.0348
III Health center II plus malaria control	1200	50.0	.0417
IV Malaria control, immunization and nutrition intervention	1450	60.0	.0414
V Health center II plus nutrition intervention and health education	1550	60.0	.0387
VI Health care system IV plus sanitation intervention	1750	70.0	.0400

Table 4.3. Anti-parasitic eradication programs

Eradication program	Financial cost (in 1000$) (1)	Reduction of morbidity (in man-days) (2)	Impact ratio (3)=(2)/(1)
Malaria	1000	2000	2
Hookworm	500	1500	3
Onchoceriasis	800	200	0.25
Schistosomiasis	500	550	1.10
Ascariasis	1500	750	0.50

In other words, it is the combination that maximizes the reduction of morbidity. *A fortiori*, any other combination will do less well in terms of reduction of morbidity. For instance, we can replace the malaria and hookworm programs by the ascariasis program, while still respecting the budget constraint. However, this particular substitution would result in an increase of morbidity by 2750 days.

Table 4.4. Ranking of eradication programs (with a given budget)

Eradication program	Impact ratio	Cumulative financial cost (in 1000$)
Hookworm	3	500
Malaria	2	1500
Schistosomiasis	1.10	2000
Ascariasis	0.50	3500
Onchocerciasis	0.25	4300

To summarize, if several competing projects satisfy the budget constraint exactly, select the project with the highest impact ratio. If alternative projects have different financial costs, but all satisfy the budget constraint, select the project with the highest impact on the objective. If a combination of interventions is to be financed by a given budget, select the interventions that have the highest impact ratios.

4.2.2. OPTIMAL CHOICE GIVEN A CERTAIN TARGET

Choosing among alternative projects

If several alternative projects can guarantee that a predetermined target will exactly be met, one has to select the alternative that minimizes costs. Let us return briefly to the second example of the previous section. If we suppose that the target consists of realizing a decrease in infant mortality of 60 per thousand, two options are feasible, *viz.* systems IV and V. The most cost-effective choice is alternative IV. Thus of the two options, it has to be the one with the *highest impact ratio*.

One has to check carefully whether the feasible alternatives reach the same targeted output. Let us illustrate this with the following example: in Heller (1975) a comparison is made between the average recurrent costs of outpatient visits at district hos-

pitals and rural health centers, in Malaysia in
1973-1974. The average cost at district hospitals
and rural health centers proved to be 2.75 and 0.84
Malaysian $, respectively. The main explanation for
the important cost advantage of the rural health
system is that rural outpatient clinics are staffed
by hospital assistants who make all initial diagnos-
ticand treatment decisions. For instance, they
treat minor ailments such as cough and fever as well
as diarrhea, roundworm infection, anemia and malaria.
Because assistants' salaries are much lower than
those of physicians, the cost of rural health clinics
is reduced *vis-à-vis* the cost of hospitals where
outpatients are seen by physicians. An additional
explanation for the low cost of the rural health
centers is that drug costs are lower because they
are stocked with inexpensive pharmaceutical products
only.

It is tempting to conclude at once that rural
health centers are more cost-effective than district
hospitals. The important question is now whether
substitution of physicians by hospital assistants
and of a whole variety of drugs by a limited range
of drugs has not lowered the quantity and quality
of health care delivered to the rural population.
Two conditions will have to be met before we can
conclude that rural health centers deliver the same
output as hospitals. *First,* the marginal product
of a physician may not be higher than that of a
well-trained hospital assistant. *Secondly,* the
limited amount of inexpensive drugs must be as
effective as the complete set of drugs available
at hospitals. In many LDC, one assumes that these
conditions are more or less met so that one assigns
health auxiliaries[1] to medical treatment of outpatients in rural health centers. The latter evidently results in low cost health care. If one can
not demonstrate that outputs are identical, the
problem is no longer that of optimal choice given
a certain target. It becomes either a problem of
optimal choice under a budget constraint or a CBA
problem!

Choosing a combination of interventions
It is also possible that one has to select a
combination of projects that reaches a specific
target and that, simultaneously, minimizes costs.
Return to the third example of the previous section.
Suppose that the target is to reduce morbidity by
3500 man-days. The procedure is then to rank again

the programs according to their impact ratios and to
select the programs starting from the top of the
ranking until the target is reached. It can be verified in Table 4.5 that the programs against malaria
and hookworm ought to be chosen. Any other combination will be suboptimal and, hence, cost more. For
instance, we can replace the hookworm program by
the programs against schistosomiasis, ascariasis
and onchocerciasis and still respect the target;
yet; it can be checked immediately that the cost of
this suboptimal combination is 2300,000 $ higher
than the cost-minimizing combination. It should be
easy to understand why the programs with the highest
impact ratios are to be favored: indeed, the higher
a ratio is, the lower the implied financial cost
for a given reduction of morbidity by one man-day.

Table 4.5. Ranking of eradication programs (with a
           given target)

Eradication program	Impact ratio	Cumulative reduction of morbidity (in man-days)
Hookworm	3	1500
Malaria	2	3500
Schistosomiasis	1.10	4050
Ascariasis	0.50	4800
Onchocerciasis	0.25	5000

4.3. CASE STUDY: A QUANTITATIVE METHOD OF ASSESSING THE HEALTH IMPACT OF DIFFERENT DISEASES IN LESS DEVELOPED COUNTRIES

4.3.1. INTRODUCTION

The study to be discussed here is that undertaken by
the Ghana Health Assessment Project Team; see Morrow
et.al. (1981). It has developed a method to estimate quantitatively the health impact of the various disease problems in Ghana. It is reasoned that
illness, disability and death are the most important
consequences of diseases. Each of these consequences
is quantified in terms of the *days of healthy life
lost* due to the diseases. This loss of healthy
days is then regarded as an approximation of the
diseases' health impact. At the same time the *benefits* of health improvement procedures are measured
by the healthy days of life that can be saved as a
result of applying these procedures.

4.3.2. THE MEASUREMENT OF HEALTHY DAYS OF LIFE LOST

The expected number of days of healthy life lost by a *patient* with a disease is

$$L = c \left[LE(A_0) - (A_d - A_0) \right] . 365.25$$
$$+ c \left[(A_d - A_0) . d_1 \right] . 365.25$$
$$+ q \left[LE(A_0) . d_2 \right] . 365.25$$
$$+ (1 - c - q) \tag{4.1}$$

where c = case fatality rate (in %)

A_0 = average age at onset of the disease

$LE(A_0)$ = expectation of life, in years, at age A_0

A_d = average age at death of those who are killed by the disease

d_1 = per cent disablement in the period from onset until death among those who die of the disease (i.e. $d_1 = 0$ % when there is no disablement, $d_1 = 100$ % for disablement equivalent to death)

d_2 = per cent disablement of those permanently disabled

q = per cent of those having the disease, who do not die of the disease but who are permanently disabled

t = average period of temporary disablement, in days

365.25 = average number of days in a year.

The loss of days is thus composed of four terms: they measure the loss due to premature deaths, disability before death, chronic disability and acute illness respectively.

The number of days lost yearly by *society* due to a particular disease is obtained as follows:

$$R = L.I \tag{4.2}$$

where I is the annual incidence of that disease per thousand population. To illustrate this procedure, the days of healthy life lost is calculated for trypanosomiasis in Ghana. The parameters are the

following (see Morrow (1981, p.75)):
$A_0=15$, $LE(A_0)=46.5$, $c=19$ %, $A_d=17$, $d_1=50$ %, $q=13.5$ %, $d_2=30$ %, $t=90$ days, $I=0.05$ %o. One can verify that the number of days of healthy life lost (R) is 195 per year per thousand population; note that the loss of healthy days due to premature death is 79.1 per cent of the total loss. In Table 4.6, we report the 25 most important diseases in Ghana in terms of days of healthy life lost.

Table 4.6. Diseases in Ghana - Ranked in order of healthy days of life lost

Rank order	Disease	Days of healthy life lost	Percent of total[+]
1	Malaria	32,600	10.2
2	Measles	23,400	7.3
3	Pneumonia (child)	18,600	5.8
4	Sickle Cell Disease	17,500	5.5
5	Malnutrition (severe)	17,500	5.5
6	Prematurity	16,800	5.2
7	Birth Injury	16,400	5.2
8	Accidents	14,900	4.7
9	Gastroenteritis	14,500	4.5
10	Tuberculosis	11,000	3.5
11	Cerebrovascular Disease	10,400	3.3
12	Pneumonia (adult)	9,100	2.9
13	Tetanus (neonatal)	6,900	2.2
14	Cirrhosis	6,600	2.1
15	Congenital Malformations	6,000	1.9
16	Complications of Pregnancy	5,900	1.8
17	Hypertension	5,100	1.6
18	Intestinal Obstruction	4,900	1.6
19	Typhoid	4,800	1.5
20	Meningitis	4,600	1.5
21	Hepatitis	4,600	1.5
22	Pertussis	4,600	1.5
23	Other Birth Diseases	4,600	1.5
24	Tetanus (adult)	4,500	1.4
25	Schistosomiasis	4,400	1.4
Total of first 25 diseases		270,200	84.9

[+]This column represents the share of each disease in the total number of days lost due to all of the 48 disease problems studied.

Source: Morrow *et al.* (1981, p.76).

4.3.3. ON THE USE OF 'DAYS OF HEALTHY LIFE LOST' IN SETTING HEALTH PRIORITIES

The calculation of the benefit measure outlined above is but one step in the cost-effectiveness analysis of health improvement procedures. Two possibilities arise further. *First,* one could focus on one disease and investigate which health improvement programs can be organized to combat this disease, how they affect the parameters in formulas (4.1) and (4.2) and how much it costs to implement them. Subsequently, the decision analysis explained in section 4.2 can be applied. Either one searches for the intervention that maximizes days of healthy life saved given a certain budget, or one selects the program that minimizes cost given a well defined target in terms of healthy days saved. *Secondly,* one can attempt to reach certain targets or objectives by devising intervention methods geared to attacking several diseases. In this case CEA directs us to choose those programs having the highest impact ratios.

In their paper Morrow *et al.* give an example of cost-effectiveness analysis. They compare the effectiveness of an immunization program against measles with that of outpatient therapy for measles. The costs of the immunization program and outpatient therapy are 20 and 72 cedis (one cedi is about one $) per thousand population, respectively. It is estimated that the benefit in terms of healthy days of life saved is 918 and 56 per cedi for the immunization program and outpatient therapy respectively. Note that the latter figures are the impact ratios of the two intervention methods. Notice that the impact ratio associated with the immunization program is 16 times as large as that of the competing program. It follows that, even if the budget would exceed 72 cedis per thousand population, the most cost-effective method is the immunization program.

4.3.4. CRITICAL COMMENTS

The authors themselves warn that much of the required information about the parameters (e.g. incidence rates, case fatality rates etc.) in formulas (4.1) and (4.2) may not be readily available from routine sources. In order to carry out their analysis for Ghana, the authors have used a variety of sources. They admit that in some cases parameters were merely

based upon a consensus. It is evident that the
benefit measure R is very sensitive to the various
parameters. Hence, one has to ascertain oneself
that the parameters are correctly estimated before
one can go ahead with the cost-effectiveness analysis. If data sources are unreliable or if certain
parameters have to be guessed, the cost-effectiveness analysis will be subject to a considerable
degree of uncertainty, of course.

A particular problem with the present approach
is that one has to attribute a single cause to the
deaths of individuals. Frequently, however, deaths
are the result of a combination of diseases. For
instance, the combination of malnutrition, malaria,
diarrhea and measles is often the cause of infant
and child death rather than one of these diseases
separately. Attributing death to one cause only
will therefore be subject to some uncertainty.

Further refinements are the following:
(i) Ideally one should use age and sex specific
parameter values pertaining to the various diseases.
The authors also raise this point but advance that
it is unlikely'that the use of age and sex specific
disease rates would make any substantial difference
to the conclusions as the onset of most of the important disease occurs over a small age range'[2].

(ii) All days lost, whether they are due to death
or disability or whether they pertain to children
or adults, have implicitly the same value to society.
It is no problem to imagine, however, that days lost
due to disability are worth less to individuals than
days lost because of death. Hence different weights
could be assigned to the days lost either due to
death or to disability. Similarly, different
weights can be given to days lost by an adult or by
a child. The reason could be that adults'days are
more valuable in terms of production than children's
days; it follows that, in that case, weights have
to tilted in favor of adults' days.

(iii) The present calculation of R also reveals
that the value of a day is independent of the time
period in which that day is lost. For instance, a
day lost at the age of 80 is as valuable as a day
lost at the age of 20. Given that most people have
some degree of preference for the present *vis-à-vis*
the future, one could assign different weights to
the days lost according to their occurrence in time.

One could make use here of the social discount rate, thus making future days less valuable than current days.

As a conclusion, we think that the concept of healthy days of life lost is a very useful and practical one. There is also no difficulty in implementing the refinements discussed above.

NOTES

[1] For further information on health auxiliaries, see Vaughan (1971) and Hu (1976).
[2] See Morrow *et al.* (1981, p.78).

Chapter Five

MULTIATTRIBUTE PROBLEM ANALYSIS

5.1. DEFINITION

Frequently, a health intervention has so many characteristics or *attributes* that it becomes difficult
to construct a unique benefit measure, as is done
by the techniques discussed previously. It may also
be that the health researcher is reluctant to melt
into one measure the information content of different attributes. Multiattribute problem analysis
(MPA) consists of procedures to decide about an optimal combination of attributes, thereby refraining
from weighting the attributes and combining them
into a single measure.

MPA can, for instance, be applied to the following problem: suppose one has to choose a project
among a number of alternative health projects to
combat tropical diseases. Each project has a number
of attributes such as the reduction of infant mortality, the reduction of adult mortality, the reduction of morbidity, the number of working days
gained, the reduction of pain and the project's
money cost. MPA will throughout the analysis respect
the six dimensions of each project. This clearly
contrasts with CBA whereby one expresses the various
costs and benefits in one monetary unit. In the
present example, one could say that MPA has the additional advantage of taking account explicitly of
such attributes as pain suffered by the ill. In CBA
this is frequently neglected because it is rather
difficult to compute the monetary equivalent of a
reduction in pain. One may also find it too tedious
to evaluate the monetary gains of decreased mortality
and morbidity and therefore turn to MPA.

MPA is different from CEA as well. Namely, in
cost-effectiveness studies, one minimizes the cost
of reaching a given target, or one maximizes(or minimizes) an objective given a certain budget. In
other words, compared to MPA, the choice problem in
CEA remains essentially unidimensional.

5.2. OBJECTIVES AND ATTRIBUTES OF HEALTH INTERVEN-
TIONS

In the literature on decisions with multiple objectives[1], one makes a distinction between an *overall*
objective, *lower-levels* objectives and *attributes*.
The first type of objective refers to an area of
concern. For instance a health intervention project may have as area of concern the improvement of
the health status of the covered population. But
this general objective gives too little information
on the specific aims of a health intervention.
Lower-level objectives have therefore to be specified such as 'reduce death' and 'reduce adult male
morbidity'. Each of these lower-level objectives
has to be further associated with attributes that
will indicate to what extent alternative health interventions meet the objectives. For example, the
death reduction objective can be associated with
the attributes infant mortality rate and adult
mortality rate, whereas the morbidity reduction objective can, for instance, be linked to the attribute 'number of workdays gained' as a result of
the health intervention. Remark that the cost of a
project may also be incorporated in the MPA as *one*
of the attributes! In MPA the issue of financial
cost is, therefore, much less important than in
CBA or CEA where budget constraints frequently play
an essential role.

As alluded to in section 5.1 a physical feeling
like pain may be an important attribute of a project.
However, it may be difficult to measure pain, unless
one is willing to construct a pain index, of course.
A reasonable alternative may be to look for a *proxy*
attribute. For instance, the number of workdays
gained could be regarded as a first (rough) approximation of the reduced amount of pain in the sense
that a workday gained represents a (painful) day
less in bed.

5.3. CHOICE PROCEDURES[2]

5.3.1. DOMINANCE

Suppose we have n types of health interventions H_i (i=1,...,n) with attributes a_i^j (j=1,...,h), where the subscript i refers to the type of intervention and superscript j to the type of attribute. Let us assume that the value to society of the health interventions depends positively on a_i^j. We can then state that, for instance, H_1 *dominates* H_2 when

$$a_1^j \geq a_2^j \quad \text{for all j}$$

$$a_1^j > a_2^j \quad \text{for some j}$$

We can continue to compare the different alternatives on a pairwise basis, until one obtains a set of *non-dominated* alternatives. The dominance technique therefore reduces the range of alternatives among which a choice has to be made. The weakness of this approach, however, is that no advice is given about the *optimal choice* to be made. Yet, a decision-maker may like this approach because he remains confronted with the different attributes up to the point of final decision.

As an example, let us take 5 possible health interventions with 4 attributes, namely reduction of the infant mortality rate (aged 0-1), reduction of the child mortality rate (aged 1-16), reduction of the adult mortality rate (aged 16+) and number of workdays gained per year per man. Below, hypothetical figures are presented in Table 5.1. We see that

Table 5.1. Search for non-dominated alternatives

Health inter-vention	Reduction in infant mortality in ‰	Reduction in child mortality in ‰	Reduction in adult mortality in ‰	Number of workdays gained per year, per man
1[+]	25	12	10	15
2	15	6	7	8
3	10	5	8	12
4	20	8	9	10
5[+]	40	10	12	14

[+]non-dominated alternatives

both health interventions 5 and 1 dominate alternatives 2, 3 and 4. It can also be seen that intervention 5 does not dominate intervention 1 because
the former performs worse in terms of the second
and fourth attribute. It is evident that the final
choice between alternatives 1 and 5 remains to be
made. That particular choice will depends upon how
the decision-maker ultimately *values* the different
attributes.

5.3.2. LEXICOGRAPHIC ORDERING

In this procedure the attributes are first *ranked*
according to importance. The procedure then determines that health intervention i is best if

$$a_i^1 > a_k^1 \quad \text{for all k (k=1,,,.,n)}$$
$$\text{where } i \neq k$$

It is possible that all health interventions do
equally well on the first attribute. One then has
to turn to the secondly ranked attribute and apply
the rule:

$$\text{select i if } a_i^2 > a_k^2 \text{ for all k (k} \neq \text{i)}$$

Again, if the alternatives are performing equally
well on the second attribute, one has to turn to
the thirdly ranked attribute etc.

Lexicographic ordering is very simple to use
and may therefore be attractive to policy-makers.
However, one has to realize that one basically
concentrates on one attribute and neglects the performance on all other attributes! To illustrate
the latter, we refer to the example of the previous
section. Suppose the reduction in child mortality
is the firstly ranked attribute. Intervention 1
will therefore be selected. This implies then that
one neglects the better performance of intervention
5 in terms of the first and third attributes!

5.3.3. SUBSTITUTION IN VALUE BETWEEN ATTRIBUTES AND THE COMPUTATION OF EQUIVALENT ALTERNATIVES

Above in 5.3.2. the preference structure was very
elementary. In this section, a procedure is analyzed whereby decision-makers are concerned with
all attributes simultaneously. To make this proce-

dure as clear as possible, we will use the example given above in 5.3.1 (see Table 5.1). The analysis there resulted in two non-dominated alternatives. Without additional information about the decision-makers' preferences, these are hard to compare, however. The way to proceed further is to look for *equivalent alternatives* whereby all attributes safe one are equalized. Thus at the end only one attribute will (or is likely to) differ so that the final choice becomes easy.

Let us start by equalizing the first attribute. The question asked is 'How much reduction in the number of work-days (per man per year) gained are you willing to accept in exchange for a further reduction in the infant mortality rate of 15 ‰?'. The answer is, say, 2. The latter figure is then the *rate of substitution* between the first and fourth attribute. In other words one is equally well off with 40 of the first attribute and 13 of the fourth attribute as with 25 and 15 of the first and fourth attribute, respectively. Table 5.2 summarizes this first stage of the procedure.

Table 5.2. Equalizing the reduction in infant mortality

Attributes	Health inter- vention 1	Health intervention 1a (=equivalent of intervention 1)	Health inter- vention 5
Reduction in infant mortality, in ‰	25	40	40
Reduction in child mortality, in ‰	12	12	10
Reduction in adult mortality, in ‰	10	10	12
Number of workdays gained per year per man	15	13	14

The next step is to equalize the second attribute. The question that can be asked here is 'How much reduction in the number of work-days (per man per year) gained are you willing to accept in exchange for a further reduction in the child mortality rate of 2 ‰?'. Suppose the rate of substitu-

tion is 0.3. The result of this step is now portrayed in Table 5.3.

Table 5.3. Equalizing the reduction in child
mortality

Attributes	Health intervention 5	Health intervention 5a (=equivalent of intervention 5)	Health intervention 1a
Reduction in infant mortality, in ‰	40	40	40
Reduction in child mortality, in ‰	10	12	12
Reduction in adult mortality, in ‰	12	12	10
Number of workdays gained per year per man	14	13.7	13

In the last step, we equalize the third attribute. Here we have to ask the question 'How much
reduction in the number of workdays (per man per
year) gained are you willing to accept in exchange
for a further reduction in the adult mortality rate
of 2 ‰?'. Assume the rate of substitution is again
0.3. The result is given in Table 5.4.

Table 5.4. Equalizing the reduction in adult
mortality

Attributes	Health intervention 1a	Health intervention 1b (=equivalent of intervention 1a)	Health intervention 5a
Reduction in infant mortality, in ‰	40	40	40
Reduction in child mortality, in ‰	12	12	12
Reduction in adult mortality, in ‰	10	12	12
Number of workdays gained per year per man	13	12.7	13.7

One can see from Table 5.4 that the choice becomes simple because only one attribute needs to be
compared. Project 5 will be selected as the best
one because its equivalent (5a) dominates the rival
project's equivalent (1b). To conclude, all that
one needs for this procedure is the willingness on
the part of the decision-maker to make explicit
trade-offs between the various attributes; another
prerequisite is, of course, that the attributes'values can be manipulated in negative and positive di-
rections.

5.4. CASE STUDY: RANKING PROGRAM ALTERNATIVES, UNDER ALTERNATIVE CRITERIA, IN RURAL JAVA

The main purpose of the research by Grosse *et al.*
(1979) is to see which cost-effective health programs can be designed, given twelve alternative per
capita budget levels, in each region of 50,000 people in rural Java. In Table 5.5 we list six alternative medical care programs that can be combined
with one out of eight possible promotional programs.
The alternative per capita budget levels are also
given in this table.

Table 5.5. Alternative programs and budget levels

Medical care programs	Promotional programs	Alternative per capita budget levels (in $)
1.Health Center (HC)	1.None	2.06
2.HC+8 Sub Health	2.Sanitation	2.50
Centers (SHC)	3.Immunization	3.00
3.HC,8 SHC,25 Village	4.Sanitation and	4.00
Health Workers(VHW)	Immunization	5.00
4.HC,8 SHC,200 VHW	5.Nutrition	7.50
5.HC,25 VHW	6.Sanitation and	10.00
6.HC, 200 VHW	Nutrition	12.50
	7.Nutrition and	15.00
	Immunization	20.00
	8.Sanitation,	25.00
	Nutrition and	30.00
	Immunization	

Source: Grosse *et al.* (1979, p.45).

At each per capita budget level[3] the impact on

disability and mortality of the 48 possible combinations is studied. In view of the fixed budget constraints, it is very well possible that a number of
combinations do not make it feasible to cover 100
per cent of the population. In order to assess the
health impacts, the authors have studied the effect
of each type of health intervention on 31 highly
prevailing diseases in rural Java. The latter means
that per intervention 31 disease profiles will be
obtained. Note that a disease profile contains such
parameters as incidence and fatality rate, days of
disability *etc.* It is evident that the disease
profile parameters may differ according to the age
cohorts considered.

In Table 5.6, we present the mortality and disability rates of the 48 alternatives when the budget
amounts to 15 $ per capita over a five year period.
Depending on which objective one wants to retain, a
different health intervention   likely to emerge as
the optimal one. For instance, the reader can verify that, if one intends to minimize total morbidity,
given the 15 $ per capita budget constraint, the
optimal choice is the combination *HC + sanitation.*
If the objective is to minimize total mortality, the
combination *HC + 200 VHW + immunization* is the most
cost-effective one.

Table 5.6. Impact on mortality and disability in
           rural Java of 48 alternative health in-
           terventions (with a budget of 15 $ per
           capita over a 5 year period)

| Combination | | Mortality (‰) | | | | | Total morbi-dity (annual dis-ability days per person) | Total morta-lity per 1000 popu-lation |
Medical care program	Promotional program	for age cohort 0-1	for age cohort 1-4	for age cohort 5-14	for age cohort 15-44	for age cohort 45+	Disability days per capita	
1	1	103.95	28.26	2.67	3.64	5.48	11.36	10.97
1	2	71.74	15.06	1.54	2.16	4.00	6.95	7.37
1	3	85.88	27.44	2.40	3.64	5.48	10.91	10.23
1	4	59.52	15.58	1.42	2.30	4.14	6.98	7.08
1	5	83.32	21.15	2.67	3.64	5.48	10.15	9.36
1	6	70.87	15.63	1.79	2.49	4.33	7.60	7.60
1	7	65.26	20.33	2.40	3.64	5.48	9.71	8.62
1	8	56.16	14.55	1.56	2.45	4.29	7.13	6.92
2	1	83.78	18.74	1.85	3.36	4.98	10.55	8.40

109

Table 5.6. (cont'd')

Combination		Mortality (‰)			Disability days per capita		Total morbidity (annual disability days per person)	Total mortality per 1000 population
Medical care program	Promotional program	for age cohort 0-1	for age cohort 1-4	for age cohort 5-14	for age cohort 15-44	for age cohort 45+		
2	2	73.77	14.41	1.40	2.31	3.99	7.50	7.18
2	3	69.16	18.27	1.69	3.36	4.98	10.11	7.84
2	4	66.03	15.12	1.38	2.41	4.10	7.49	7.08
2	5	67.89	13.66	1.85	3.36	4.98	9.46	7.21
2	6	73.21	15.41	1.64	2.56	4.27	7.97	7.48
2	7	53.26	13.19	1.69	3.36	4.98	9.01	6.66
2	8	63.20	14.72	1.50	2.52	4.23	7.59	7.03
3	1	84.00	21.06	2.02	3.36	4.95	10.51	8.83
3	2	72.83	15.63	1.56	2.42	4.10	7.80	7.44
3	3	68.27	20.52	1.82	3.36	4.95	10.07	8.22
3	4	65.12	16.15	1.52	2.51	4.19	7.76	7.30
3	5	67.36	15.73	2.02	3.36	4.95	9.41	7.58
3	6	72.90	16.57	1.75	2.63	4.33	8.18	7.71
3	7	51.64	15.18	1.82	3.36	4.95	8.97	6.97
3	8	63.01	15.92	1.61	2.60	4.30	7.84	7.27
4	1	64.49	12.68	1.54	3.10	4.43	9.35	6.62
4	2	77.74	17.50	1.77	2.68	4.27	8.54	7.93
4	3	54.89	13.77	1.48	3.15	4.53	9.15	6.52
4	4	72.15	17.83	1.73	2.73	4.33	8.48	7.82
4	5	65.00	14.03	1.80	3.22	4.67	9.15	7.05
4	6	77.97	18.36	1.88	2.80	4.42	8.76	8.15
4	7	57.39	14.78	1.73	3.25	4.73	9.01	6.94
4	8	70.98	17.97	1.79	2.78	4.40	8.52	7.85
5	1	85.34	21.35	2.06	3.40	5.05	10.54	8.97
5	2	67.17	13.11	1.36	2.21	3.89	7.11	6.78
5	3	68.90	20.74	1.83	3.40	5.05	10.10	8.32
5	4	57.98	13.88	1.30	2.32	4.02	7.13	6.64
5	5	68.23	15.92	2.06	3.40	5.05	9.44	7.70
5	6	68.17	14.69	1.62	2.49	4.21	7.69	7.23
5	7	51.79	15.31	1.83	3.40	5.05	9.00	7.05
5	8	56.04	13.83	1.44	2.45	4.17	7.27	6.67
6	1	67.18	13.36	1.60	3.21	4.72	9.44	6.94
6	2	75.07	16.13	1.66	2.61	4.26	8.21	7.63
6	3	50.99	12.83	1.38	3.21	4.72	9.00	6.31
6	4	68.45	16.53	1.61	2.66	4.33	8.16	7.49
6	5	58.28	11.47	1.69	3.25	4.78	8.77	6.47
6	6	75.35	17.25	1.81	2.75	4.44	8.50	7.90
6	7	48.89	12.56	1.59	3.28	4.84	8.63	6.36
6	8	67.03	16.74	1.68	2.73	4.41	8.23	7.53

Source: Grosse *et al.* (1979, Appendix F).

Frequently, however, decision-makers have more than one criterion to which they are sensitive. Suppose indeed that they want to take account of, say, two attributes, *viz.* total morbidity and total mortality. If they apply the *dominance* approach, they will obtain as a result of the analysis a list of non-dominated alternatives. The solution of this multiattribute problem, using the data in Table 5.6, is portrayed in Table 5.7. The final choice of a single best alternative among the six non-dominated alternatives will further depend upon the value judgments or preferences of the decision-makers.

Table 5.7. Non-dominated alternatives according to the attributes total morbidity and total mortality

Total morbidity	Total mortality	Program alternatives
6.95	7.37	HC, Sanitation
9.00	6.31	HC, 200 VHW, Immunization
6.98	7.08	HC, Sanitation, Immunization
7.11	6.78	HC, 25 VHW, Sanitation
7.13	6.64	HC, 25 VHW, Sanitation, Immunization
8.63	6.36	HC, 200 VHW, Nutrition, Immunization

Source: Grosse *et al.* (1979, p.60).

NOTES

[1] See Keeney and Raiffa (1976, p.32).
[2] *Ibidem* (ch.3).
[3] The different levels are maintained over a five year period.

Chapter Six

LINEAR PROGRAMMING

6.1. DEFINITION

Programming is defined by Baumol (1977, p.76) as
'the mathematical method for the analysis and compu-
tation of optimal decisions which do not violate the
limitations imposed by inequality side conditions'.
One speaks of *linear* programming (LP) if, in the objective function and constraints, the variables are
multiplied by constants and added together. The
common element with the evaluation methods discussed
up to now is that one also maximizes or minimizes
some objective by means of an optimal allocation of
resources or inputs. A specific characteristic is
that in LP one uses *inequality* constraints; in problems where an objective is maximized subject to certain constraints, for instance, this feature of LP
implies that maximum available resources do not have
to be exhausted.

6.2. FORMULATION OF A LP PROBLEM

The general formulation[1] of a LP problem is:

$$\text{optimize (maximize or minimize)} \quad \sum_{j=1}^{n} w_j x_j \qquad (6.1)$$

$$\text{subject to} \quad \sum_{j=1}^{n} a_{ji} x_j \ (\leq, \geq, =) r_i \quad i=1,\ldots,m \qquad (6.2)$$

$$\text{and} \quad x_j \geq 0 \qquad\qquad j=1,\ldots,n \qquad (6.3)$$

When the LP problem is a *maximization* problem,
(6.1) is called the *maximand*; x_j is decision variable j whereas w_j is the coefficient of x_j that re-

112

presents the contribution per unit of x_j to the
maximand. Expression (6.2) refers to the *structural
constraints* in which a_{ij} and r_i are constants. Note
that each structural constraint is associated with
only one sign in $(\leq, >, =)$. Finally, (6.3) refers to
the *nonnegative* constraints.

If the LP problem is a *minimization* problem,
(6.1) can be referred to as the *minimand*. The coefficient w_j is then the contribution per unit of x_j
to the minimand. As before (6.2) and (6.3) are the
structural constraints and nonnegativity constraints
respectively. Note finally that both the maximand
and the minimand can be called *objective functions*.

LP may be very useful in deciding upon the optimal allocation of resources in health projects.
For instance, if we look upon the organisation of a
health project as a *maximization* problem, the x
variables may refer to health inputs such as drugs,
vaccinations, labor time of health workers, midwives,
nurses, physicians etc. The w_j weights could be expressed, for instance, in terms of lives saved. The
restrictions could contain, say, an overall budget
constraint for the health project and separate restrictions on health inputs. The example just given
may be easily converted into a *minimization* problem.
The problem to be solved could then be to minimize
the cost of the health inputs subject to the minimum
achievement of certain health goals such as a minimum number of lives of infants and adults to be
saved.

6.3. GRAPHICAL SOLUTION FOR A LP PROBLEM WITH TWO CHOICE VARIABLES

The solution for problems with two choice variables
can be depicted rather easily on a graph. Let us
first present a solution for the organisation of a
health project seen as a *maximization* problem:

maximize $\qquad 163\ x_1 + 100\ x_2$ $\qquad\qquad$ (6.4)

subject to $\qquad 20\ x_1 + 5\ x_2 \leq 200$ $\qquad\qquad$ (6.5)

$\qquad\qquad\qquad\qquad x_1 \leq 5$ $\qquad\qquad$ (6.6)

$\qquad\qquad\qquad\qquad x_2 \leq 30$ $\qquad\qquad$ (6.7)

$\qquad\qquad x_1 \geq 0 \qquad x_2 \geq 0$ $\qquad\qquad$ (6.8)

Figure 6.1. Graphical solution of a maximization problem

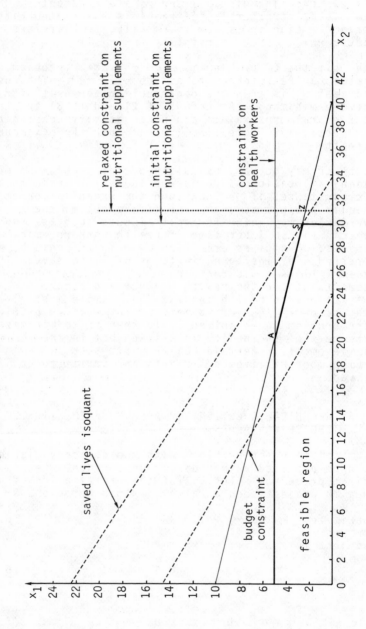

In (6.4), the variables x_1 and x_2 denote health workers (in man-years) and nutritional supplements (*e.g.* milk in tons) respectively. The coefficients in the maximand represent contributions to lives saved in the region where the health project will be set up. Restriction (6.5) is a budget constraint in which the coefficients represent the prices of the two health inputs. Restrictions (6.6) and (6.7) refer to constraints on the maximum available inputs in the region, whereas (6.8) represents the nonnegative constraints.

The solution is presented in Figure 6.1. The area contoured by the bold lines is called the *feasible region*. The latter contains all feasible solutions to the LP problem. The dashed lines represent the *saved live isoquants*[2]. It can be seen that at point S an improvement in saved lives is no longer possible. Hence, the optimum is represented by *corner* S of the feasible region. One can verify that the number of lives saved at the optimum is approximately 3407. The optimum dictates that all available nutritional supplements are to be used whereas only 2.5 man-years of health workers are needed.

We now turn to the graphical solution of a *minimization* problem with two choice variables. Suppose the problem at hand is that of minimizing the money cost of an anti-malaria campaign that uses two types of insecticides. The requirements are that a minimum number of lives has to be saved and that a minimum number of mosquitos has to be exterminated. This hypothetical program is as follows

minimize $\qquad$ $15 x_1 + 10 x_2$ $\qquad\qquad$ (6.9)

subject to $\qquad$ $200 x_1 + 100 x_2 \geq 1600$ $\qquad$ (6.10)

$\qquad\qquad$ $1000 x_1 + 200 x_2 \geq 14000$ $\qquad$ (6.11)

Requirement (6.10) implies that a minimum of 1600 lives have to be saved whereas requirement (6.11) imposes the eradication of at least 14000 mosquitos. In Figure 6.2, the graphical solution is presented. The set of feasible solutions is now to be found to the right of the bold lines. In the present case, the dashed lines refer to *isocost curves*[3]. It can be seen that the optimum occurs at point T. At the latter point, no reductions in money cost are possible without leaving the feasible region. The inputs

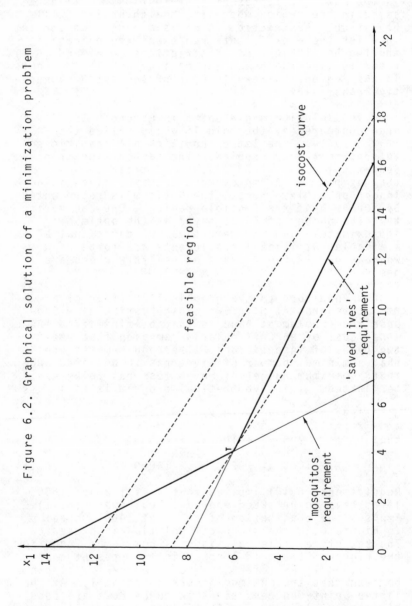

Figure 6.2. Graphical solution of a minimization problem

Linear programming

to be allocated at T amount to 6 and 4 of x_1 and x_2, respectively. The minimum cost is therefore equal to 130.

6.4. SHADOW PRICES

The solution of the maximization problem in the previous section implied that the constraints on nutritional supplements and on the budget were *binding*; the latter means that both the budget and the available nutritional supplements are completely utilized. The constraint on health workers could be seen to be *nonbinding*, meaning that the demand is strictly less than the available supply of health workers. Suppose now that we relax the constraint on nutritional supplements, namely $x_2 < 31$ instead of $x_2 < 30$. In Figure 6.1 the constraint (6.7) moves to the right, entailing an increased value for the objective represented by point Z. Again, x_2 is fully utilized whereas 2.2 man-years of health workers are needed. The quantity of saved lives is approximately 3459 at Z whereas it is 3407 at S. This increase in saved lives, namely 52, is due to a unitary increment of the constant at the right-hand side of (6.7). We can now say that 52 is the *shadow price* of nutritional supplements. In other words the shadow price of a resource is the change in the value of the objective as the available quantity of that resource increases by one unit. We can also state that the shadow price gives us information about the opportunity we loose in not being able to employ additional resource units because of a strict resource constraint.

In the event of a resource with a nonbinding constraint, the shadow price is zero. Indeed, in that case, the solution of the LP problem is independent of the available supply of that resource since, at the optimum, the supply exceeds the demand for this resource. So, increasing the available quantity of that resource would certainly not result in an improvement of the objective, hence entailing a zero shadow price.

6.5. PROBLEMS IN USING LP FOR HEALTH PROJECTS

Firstly, problems in health care evaluations are likely to be much more complicated than the simple examples given above[4]. In practice, most LP problems are likely to have many constraints. For instance, in the case of optimizing the output of a health project, there may be constraints on the quantities of different categories of health personnel and on the use of various health determinants such as education, sanitation, nutrition, family planning *etc*. Solution techniques such as the *simplex method* exist now to handle more complicated LP problems[5]. The reader has noticed that an optimal solution to an LP problem occurs at a corner of the feasible region. The simplex method essentially calculates the values of the objective function at the corners of the feasible region in order to select the corner that corresponds to the optimal value of the objective.

Secondly, it may be possible that either the objective function or the constraints, or both, are nonlinear, so that the application of *non-linear* programming may become necessary. Furthermore, one of the assumptions of LP is that all activities assume continuous values. It frequently happens that choices require integer solutions: this is especially true if one has to choose an optimal number of project buildings or vehicles, for instance. In the latter case, one may want to use *integer* programming.

Thirdly, it is evident that one needs careful information about prices and the way constraints are to be formulated. Moreover, one has to agree upon the objective. In some cases, the health researcher would want to consider multiple objectives rather than a single objective. The latter problem can be solved by means of *goal* programming which is a variant of LP[6].

Despite the warnings concerning the use of linear programming, it has to be recognized that programming in general is a valuable technique for tackling choice problems in health care intervention. The requirement is, once again, that one should have correct information about the specification of constraints and that one should agree upon the formulation of the objective(s). Nowadays, various computer algorithms are available, even for micro-computers, which eventually will allow the health researcher to use programming techniques successfully.

NOTES

[1] See also Budnick, Mojena and Vollman (1977, pp.108-109).
[2] In an isoquant, the various alternative combinations of inputs are depicted that secure an identical output. In the present case, the output is the amount of lives saved.
[3] An isocost curve represents various combinations of inputs that lead to an identical financial cost.
[4] See *e.g.* Dunlop (1982).
[5] See Baumol (1977, ch.5) for a thorough description of this method.
[6] See Budnick, Mojena and Vollman (1977, pp. 351-366).

Chapter Seven

REGRESSION ANALYSIS

7.1. DEFINITION

Regression analysis (RA) is a statistical method
that is used to estimate the relationship between a
dependent variable and one or more independent variables. RA can be applied to investigate a wide
range of issues. Let us mention a few possibilities.
As is already demonstrated in the first chapter, RA
is useful to the health researcher who is interested
in finding determinants of health status variables.
RA can also be used to estimate the demand for various types of health care. Another fruitful application is the estimation of cost curves; one can estimate, for instance, the effect of the amount of personnel, the number of beds and the hospital case-mix
on the hospital costs. In this chapter, we will explain the basics of the simple and multiple linear
regression model.

7.2. THE SIMPLE LINEAR REGRESSION MODEL

7.2.1. HOW TO ESTIMATE THE RELATIONSHIP BETWEEN TWO VARIABLES?

The simplest relationship to be treated by RA is the
following one

$$y = \beta_1 + \beta_2 x + u \tag{7.1}$$

where y and x are the *dependent* and *independent* or
explanatory variable, respectively. The coefficients
β_1 and β_2 are the *intercept* and *slope* of the relationship, respectively. The u term in (7.1) refers to a
disturbance or *random term*. The latter indicates
that other influences, not captured by x, are at

work in determining y. Yet, these influences are unpredictable and unobservable so that we remain basically interested in the relationship between y and x. The purpose of RA now is to estimate the *population parameters* β_1 and β_2 on the basis of a number of sample observations on y and x. These observations may be time series or cross-section data. We will represent n observations as dots in a scatter diagram (see Figure 7.1).

In RA the *least squares criterion* is used in order to estimate β_1 and β_2. This criterion consists of minimizing the sum of the squared deviations between the observed y's and the explained y's (denoted henceforth by ŷ). In other words, RA aims at obtaining a fitted line that is as close as possible to the observations. We may further write that

$$\hat{y} = \hat{\beta}_1 + \hat{\beta}_2 x \qquad\qquad (7.2)$$

where $\hat{\beta}_1$ and $\hat{\beta}_2$ refer to the estimated parameters. Eq.(7.2) is also the formula of the *regression line*, depicted in Figure 7.1 as the straight line. The sum of squared deviations between y and ŷ is written as follows:

$$\sum_{i=1}^{n} e_i^2 = \sum_{i=1}^{n} (y_i - \hat{y}_i)^2$$

$$= \sum_{i=1}^{n} (y_i - \hat{\beta}_1 - \hat{\beta}_2 x_i)^2 \qquad\qquad (7.3)$$

where the subscript i refers to the i-th observation and e_i is the *residual* i or the deviation between y_i and $\hat{y}_i$.

Following the least squares criterion, we have to select $\hat{\beta}_1$ and $\hat{\beta}_2$ such that (7.3) is minimized. Therefore we need to differentiate (7.3) with respect to $\hat{\beta}_1$ and $\hat{\beta}_2$ and set the results equal to 0. The results of this differentiation procedure are:

$$\frac{\partial}{\partial \hat{\beta}_1} (\sum_{i=1}^{n} e_i^2) = -2 \sum_{i=1}^{n} (y_i - \hat{\beta}_1 - \hat{\beta}_2 x_i) = 0 \quad (7.4)$$

$$\frac{\partial}{\partial \hat{\beta}_2} (\sum_{i=1}^{n} e_i^2) = -2 \sum_{i=1}^{n} x_i (y_i - \hat{\beta}_1 - \hat{\beta}_2 x_i) = 0 \quad (7.5)$$

Figure 7.1. Scatter diagram

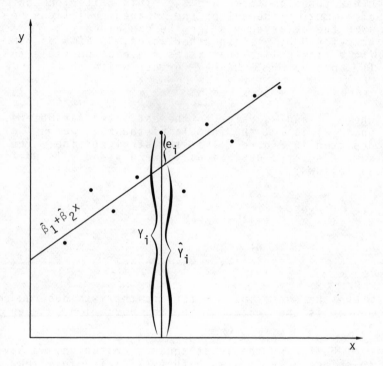

After rearranging (7.4) and (7.5), we obtain the following two *normal* equations:

$$\sum_{i=1}^{n} y_i = \hat{\beta}_1 n + \hat{\beta}_2 \sum_{i=1}^{n} x_i \qquad (7.6)$$

$$\sum_{i=1}^{n} x_i y_i = \hat{\beta}_1 \sum_{i=1}^{n} x_i + \hat{\beta}_2 \sum_{i=1}^{n} x_i^2 \qquad (7.7)$$

The intercept can be derived from (7.6), namely:

$$\hat{\beta}_1 = \bar{y} - \hat{\beta}_2 \bar{x} \qquad (7.8)$$

where $\bar{y}$ and $\bar{x}$ denote the average of the observations on y and x respectively. If we insert (7.8) into (7.7), we can obtain, after rearranging terms, an expression for the slope:

$$\hat{\beta}_2 = \frac{\sum_{i=1}^{n} x_i y_i - \bar{y} \sum_{i=1}^{n} x_i}{\sum_{i=1}^{n} x_i^2 - \bar{x} \sum_{i=1}^{n} x_i} \qquad (7.9)$$

Eq.(7.9) is also called the *estimator* of the slope.

7.2.2. EXPLANATORY POWER OF THE REGRESSION

We know that the application of the least squares criterion guarantees a best fit. The quality of this fit can now be measured by the *coefficient of determination* R^2. The latter is defined as

$$R^2 = 1 - \frac{\text{var } e_i}{\text{var } y_i} \qquad (7.10)$$

where the nominator and denominator in the second term on the right-hand side of (7.10) are the variances of the residuals and of the dependent variable y, respectively; namely,

$$\text{var } e_i = \frac{\sum_{i=1}^{n} e_i^2}{n} \quad \text{and} \quad \text{var } y_i = \frac{\sum_{i=1}^{n} (y_i - \bar{y})^2}{n} \qquad (7.11)[1]$$

The R^2 reflects the *explained* variance of the dependent variable. If, for instance, R^2 assumes a value of 0.90, one says that 90 per cent of the total variation of y is explained by the regression equation.

Frequently, one uses the *unbiased* estimators of the variances of e_i and y_i in order to calculate the coefficient of determination[2]. One then obtains:

$$\bar{R}^2 = 1 - \frac{\sum\limits_{i=1}^{n} e_i^2 / n-k}{\sum\limits_{i=1}^{n} (y_i - \bar{y})^2 / n-1} \qquad (7.12),$$

where k is the number of coefficients to be estimated. One refers to $\bar{R}^2$ as the coefficient of determination adjusted for degrees of freedom[3]. It can be seen that the $\bar{R}^2$ adjusts for the number of independent variables whereas R^2 does not.

7.2.3. EXAMPLE

Let us study the following relationship:

$$EXP = \beta_1 + \beta_2 \ GNP + u$$

where EXP = Public expenditure on health per capita ($)
GNP = Gross National Product per capita ($).

This equation will be estimated using cross-section data of 1976 for 65 developing countries. The data are listed in Table 7.1. It is expected that β_2 will be positive so as to convey that as a country becomes wealthier it will devote more public resources to health care.

Using the data we derive the following[4]:

$$\sum_{i=1}^{65} x_i y_i = 280,460 \qquad \bar{y} = 6.09231$$

$$\sum_{i=1}^{65} x_i = 29,390 \qquad \bar{x} = 452.154$$

Regression analysis

Table 7.1. Data for EXP and GNP in 1976

Country	EXP	GNP	Country	EXP	GNP
Bangladesh	1	110	Uganda	3	240
Lao P.R.	1	90	Sudan	2	290
Ethiopia	1	100	Angola	3	330
Mali	2	100	Indonesia	1	240
Nepal	1	120	Togo	3	260
Somalia	3	110	Egypt	8	280
Burundi	1	120	Cameroon	3	290
Chad	1	120	Yemen P.R.	2	280
Rwanda	1	110	China P.R.	5	410
Zaire	1	140	Honduras	10	390
Burma	1	120	Nigeria	3	380
Malawi	2	140	Thailand	2	380
India	2	150	Philippines	3	410
Mozambique	1	170	Zambia	13	440
Niger	1	160	Congo P.R.	10	520
Afghanistan	1	160	Papua New Guinea	14	490
Pakistan	1	170	Rhodesia	8	550
Sierra Leone	3	200	El Salvador	7	490
Benin	3	130	Morocco	7	540
Guinea	4	150	Bolivia	6	390
Haiti	1	200	Albania	7	540
Central African Republic	2	230	Korea D.R.	1	470
			Ivory Coast	9	610
Kenya	4	240	Jordan	7	610
Mauritania	3	340	Malaysia	13	860
Colombia	6	630	Algeria	13	990
Ecuador	7	640	Turkey	6	990
Guatemala	6	630	Mexico	9	1090
Nicaragua	11	750	Jamaica	41	1070
Mongolia	11	860	Panama	19	1310
Dominic.Republic	11	780	Uruguay	12	1390
Peru	10	800	Iraq	8	1390
Tunisia	15	840			
Cuba	19	860			

Source: EXP and GNP are taken from World Bank
(1980a, pp.75-77) and World Bank (1977).

$$\sum_{i=1}^{65} x_i^2 = 20,791,300$$

Using this information in (7.8) and (7.9) results in
the following coefficient estimates:

125

$$\hat{\beta}_1 = -0.0192 \qquad \hat{\beta}_2 = 0.0135$$

Noting that $\sum\limits_{i=1}^{65} e_i^2 = 1288.78$ and $\sum\limits_{i=1}^{65} (y_i - \bar{y})^2 =$ 2659.45, it can be derived that $\bar{R}^2 = 0.507$. Hence about 51 per cent of the variance of EXP is explained by the regression equation

$$EXP = -0.0192 + 0.0135 \; GNP.$$

7.3. THE MULTIPLE LINEAR REGRESSION MODEL[5]

7.3.1. LEAST SQUARES ESTIMATION OF COEFFICIENTS

Suppose we have a relationship of the form

$$y_i = \beta_1 + \beta_2 x_{2i} + \beta_3 x_{3i} + \beta_4 x_{4i} + \ldots + \beta_k x_{ki} + u_i \qquad (7.13),$$

with $i = 1, \ldots, n$ (observations). One can see that relationship (7.13) contains $k-1$ explanatory variables. The matrix formulation of (7.13) is

$$Y = XB + U \qquad (7.14),$$

where Y is a $n \times 1$ vector of values of the dependent variable, X is $n \times k$ matrix of the independent variables (including a vector of ones[6]), B is a $k \times 1$ vector of coefficients (including β_1) and U is a $n \times 1$ vector of random terms.

The expression for the regression line, similar to (7.2) is

$$\hat{Y} = X\hat{B}$$

where $\hat{Y}$ and $\hat{B}$ represent the vector of explained $\hat{Y}_i$'s and the vector of estimated coefficients $\hat{\beta}_j (j=1, \ldots, k)$ respectively.

The sum of squared deviations between Y and $\hat{Y}$ is now:

$$E'E = (Y - X\hat{B})'(Y - X\hat{B})$$

$$= Y'Y - 2\hat{B}'X'Y + \hat{B}'X'X\hat{B}$$

where E is a column vector of $n \times 1$ residuals.

We now have to find values for $\hat{B}$ such that $E'E$ is minimized. We next set the partial derivative of $E'E$ with respect to $\hat{B}$ equal to 0:

$$\frac{\partial E'E}{\partial \hat{B}} = -2X'Y + 2X'X\hat{B} = 0 \qquad (7.15)$$

From (7.15) we can derive the formula of the least squares estimators:

$$\hat{B} = (X'X)^{-1} X'Y \qquad (7.16)$$

7.3.2. VARIANCE-COVARIANCE MATRIX OF THE COEFFICIENTS[7]

Regarding the disturbance terms, the following assumptions are made in RA:

(i) The expected value of u_i is 0, namely[8]

$$E(U) = 0 \qquad (7.17)$$

(ii) The variance-covariance matrix of the random terms u_i, $V(U)$, is diagonal:

$$V(U) = E(UU') = \sigma^2 I \qquad (7.18)$$

where σ^2 is a constant (to be estimated) and I is a nxn identity matrix. Eq.(7.18) implies that all covariance terms in $V(U)$ are zero; the latter means that the disturbances in different observations are assumed to be independent.

We are now equipped to find the variance-covariance matrix of the regression coefficients. The latter are also stochastic because they depend upon the stochastic variable Y. This variance-covariance matrix is defined as

$$V(\hat{B}) = E\{\hat{B}-E(\hat{B})\}\{\hat{B}-E(\hat{B})\}' \qquad (7.19)$$

In view of (7.14), (7.16) and (7.17), we have that

$$E(\hat{B}) = E\{(X'X)^{-1}X'Y\}$$

$$= E\{(X'X)^{-1}X'(XB+U)\}$$

$$= E\{(X'X)^{-1}(X'X)B+(X'X)^{-1}X'U\}$$

$$= B+(X'X)^{-1}X'E(U)$$

$$E(\hat{B}) = B \qquad (7.20)$$

Equation (7.20) shows that with the assumptions made above, the estimation of B is unbiased: i.e. its expectation equals the vector of population parameters. This is an important statistical property.

Using (7.14), (7.18) and (7.20), we can rewrite (7.19) as

$$V(\hat{B}) = E\{(X'X)^{-1}X'(XB+U)-B\}\{(X'X)^{-1}X'(XB+U)-B\}'$$

$$= E\{(X'X)^{-1}X'UU'X(X'X)^{-1}\}$$

$$= \sigma^2(X'X)^{-1} \qquad (7.21)$$

From (7.21), we can derive that the variance of any regression coefficient is equal to σ^2 times the appropriate diagonal element of the matrix $(X'X)^{-1}$. The *standard errors* of the coefficients are obtained by taking the square root of the diagonal elements of (7.21). Of course, if we actually want to compute the standard errors, we need to have an estimate of the unknown σ^2. We now state without proof[9] that

$$\hat{\sigma}^2 = E'E/n-k$$

can be used as an unbias estimator of the unknown variance of the disturbance terms. The square root of $\hat{\sigma}^2$ is called the *standard error of estimate*; it represents the average error made in the regression.

7.3.3. CONFIDENCE INTERVALS

We further assume that the random variable U follows a *normal distribution*. Hence, Y has also a normal distribution. The latter implies that the coefficients $\hat{B}$ are also normally distributed since they are linearly related to Y. We can then standardize $\hat{\beta}_j$ in the following way

$$z_j = \frac{\hat{\beta}_j - \beta_j}{\sqrt{V(\hat{B})_{jj}}} \qquad j=1,\ldots,k \qquad (7.22)$$

where $V(\hat{B})_{jj}$ is the j-th diagonal element of the variance-covariance matrix of the regression coefficients. z_j is a normally distributed variable with mean 0 and variance 1.

When we replace subsequently σ^2 by $\hat{\sigma}^2$ in $V(\hat{\beta})_{jj}$ of (7.22), it turns out that the standardized $\hat{\beta}_j$ follows a t-distribution; namely

$$t_j = \frac{\hat{\beta}_j - \beta_j}{\sqrt{\hat{\sigma}^2 (X'X)_{jj}^{-1}}} \qquad j=1,\ldots,k \qquad (7.23)$$

has a t-distribution with n-k degrees of freedom[10]. Note that $(X'X)_{jj}^{-1}$ is the j-th diagonal element of the $(X'X)^{-1}$ matrix.

If $t_{\alpha/2}$ and $-t_{\alpha/2}$ refer to the t-values[11] that leave $\alpha/2$ per cent of the distribution in the upper tail and $\alpha/2$ per cent of the distribution in the lower tail, respectively, we can write that

$$\Pr(-t_{\alpha/2} < t < t_{\alpha/2}) = 1 - \frac{\alpha}{100} \qquad (7.24),$$

where Pr denotes probability. Substituting (7.23) in (7.24), we have

$$\Pr\left(-t_{\alpha/2} < \frac{\hat{\beta}_j - \beta_j}{\sqrt{\hat{\sigma}^2 (X'X)_{jj}^{-1}}} < t_{\alpha/2}\right) = 1 - \frac{\alpha}{100} \qquad j=1,\ldots,k$$

From the latter expression, we can derive that the $(1-\alpha/100)$ *confidence interval* for the population parameter β_j is

$$\beta_j = \hat{\beta}_j \pm t_{\alpha/2} \sqrt{\hat{\sigma}^2 (X'X)_{jj}^{-1}} \qquad (7.25).$$

The latter expression thus indicates that there is a chance of $(1-\alpha/100)$ that the true β_j lies in the interval given by the right-hand side of (7.25).

7.3.4. HYPOTHESIS TESTING

A *two-sided test* can be performed by inspecting whether the confidence interval (7.25) contains the hypothesis formulated. A hypothesis frequently tested is

the null hypothesis: $H_0 : \beta_j = 0$

against the alternative: $H_A : \beta_j \neq 0$

If the value of zero is not contained in the interval (7.25), one rejects the null hypothesis at the α per cent *significance level*. Note that we only make a α per cent error by not accepting the null hypothesis. Typically α is chosen to be 5 or 1 per cent.

Suppose that one expects a coefficient to be positive. In that case the alternative hypothesis may be formulated differently. One then has a *one-sided test*:

the null hypothesis: $H_0 : \beta_j = 0$

against the alternative: $H_A : \beta_j > 0$

In this test,

$$t_j = \frac{\hat{\beta}_j}{\sqrt{\hat{\sigma}^2 (X'X)^{-1}_{jj}}} \qquad (7.26)$$

has a probability of $(1-\alpha/100)$ per cent to assume values below t_α. If t_j does exceed t_α, we may reject the null hypothesis with a confidence level of $(1-\alpha/100)$.

7.3.5. EXAMPLE

We postulate the following relationship:

$$CONTRA = \beta_1 + \beta_2 PHY + \beta_3 LIT + u$$

where CONTRA = percentage of married women using contraceptives
PHY = population per physician
LIT = adult literacy rate (per cent).
By means of data for 18 developing countries, we will estimate the parameters of this relationship. Note that CONTRA is from 1979 whereas the data on PHY and LIT pertain to 1977. It is expected that $\hat{\beta}_2$ will be negative. The reasoning is as follows. A high value for PHY reflects a low availability of medical personnel. One can put forward the hypothesis that the lower the availability of physicians, the less information about contraceptives and the less prescriptions will be given to married women. The latter explains our hypothesis that $\hat{\beta}_2 < 0$. The coefficient $\hat{\beta}_3$ is expected to be positive. The explanation is the following. The adult literacy

rate is a proxy for the literacy rate among women. The higher the literacy rate now, the more women are likely to understand the purpose of the use of contraceptives, hence the hypothesis is that $\beta_3 > 0$.

The data are listed in Table 7.2. The results of applying (7.16) are

$$\hat{\beta}_1 = -7.7966 \qquad \hat{\beta}_2 = -0.000194 \qquad \hat{\beta}_3 = 0.6022$$

The variance-covariance matrix of the coefficients is

$$\hat{\sigma}^2 (X'X)^{-1} = \begin{bmatrix} 156.356 & -0.00406 & -1.88222 \\ -0.00406 & 0.000000228 & 0.0000401 \\ -1.88222 & 0.0000401 & 0.0256967 \end{bmatrix}$$

By taking the square root of the diagonal elements of the latter matrix, we obtain the standard errors of the coefficients: these are 12.5043, 0.000478 and 0.1603 for $\hat{\beta}_1$, $\hat{\beta}_2$ and $\hat{\beta}_3$ respectively. The $\bar{R}^2$ of the regression equation is 0.5389.

Let us now perform a two-sided test on whether $\beta_2 = 0$. Applying (7.25), the 95 per cent confidence interval and noting that $t_{0.025} = 2.131$ (at 15 degrees of freedom), we have

$$\beta_2 = -0.000194 \pm 2.131 \times 0.000478$$

or

$$-0.001213 < \beta_2 < 0.0008246$$

We see that 0 is contained in the interval, hence we may accept the null hypothesis that the true parameter β_2 is zero; in other words, we may reject the hypothesis that the number of physicians influences the use of contraceptives.

We will next perform the following one-sided test:

the null hypothesis: $\beta_3 = 0$

against the alternative: $\beta_3 > 0$

Applying (7.26), we have

$$t_3 = \frac{0.6022}{0.1603} = 3.7567$$

The latter value exceeds $t_{0.05}$ (at 15 degrees of freedom) that is equal to 1.753. Hence, we can reject
the null hypothesis with a 95 per cent confidence
level. We may thus conclude that literacy has a
statistically significant impact on the use of contraceptives.

Table 7.2. Data for CONTRA in 1979 and PHY and LIT
in 1977

Country	CONTRA	PHY	LIT
Bangladesh	2	12690	26
Nepal	4	35900	19
India	23	3630	36
Sri Lanka	41	6700	85
Pakistan	6	3780	24
Kenya	7	11630	50
Indonesia	27	13670	62
Egypt	17	1050	44
Zimbabwe	14	7030	74
Thailand	39	8220	84
Philippines	37	2810	75
Paraguay	16	2190	84
Tunisia	21	3580	62
Korea Rep. of	49	1980	93
Costa Rica	64	1390	90
Mexico	40	1260	81
Iran	23	2560	50
Hong Kong	79	1180	90

Source: World Bank (1982).

7.4. SOME REFINEMENTS

7.4.1. TRANSFORMATION OF VARIABLES

Double-log transformation
    Above, we have discussed relationships that
were of the linear type. It is evident that phenomena may not always be captured in a linear framework. Suppose we study the effect of nutrients on
the number of healthy days of life. It may be assumed that the effect of additional nutrients de-
clines as one approaches an adequate health status
(measured by healthy days of life); in that case,
one may speak of a decreasing marginal effect of
nutrients. For this particular relation, a *non-
linear* specification[12] will be appropriate, namely

$$y = \beta_1 \, x^{\beta_2} \qquad\qquad (7.27)$$

where y and x refer to healthy days and nutrients, respectively, and where[13] $\beta_2 < 1$. Taking logarithms of (7.27), we obtain

$$\ln y = \tilde{\beta}_1 + \beta_2 \ln x \qquad\qquad (7.28)$$

where $\tilde{\beta}_1 = \ln \beta_1$. The least squares method can be used to estimate (7.28), by considering directly the transformed variables.

The relation between y and x (with $\beta_2 < 1$) can be depicted in Figure 7.2 as the continuous curve. In a relationship were x has an increasing marginal effect on y, β_2 will be larger than 1; it is represented in the same figure by the dashed curve.

Figure 7.2. Double-log transformation

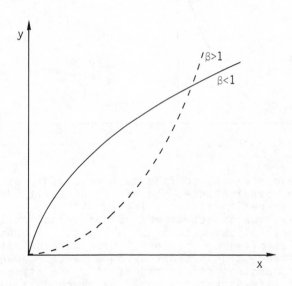

Logarithmic reciprocal transformation
The specification of this transformation is the following:

$$y = e^{\alpha - \frac{\beta}{x}}$$

or

$$\ln y = \alpha - \frac{\beta}{x}$$

This function has the property that y goes to zero as x tends to zero and that y tends to e^{α} as x goes to infinity. It can also be shown that to the left of $x = \beta/2$ (called the inflection point) the slope[14] of this function increases whereas it decreases to the right of this point. The shape of this function is revealed in Figure 7.3.

Figure 7.3. Logarithmic reciprocal transformation

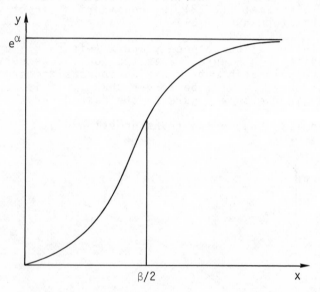

One may expect to find such relationships when studying, for instance, the effect of health determinants on health status. Indeed, it is possible that, say, the impact of medical personnel on life expectancy follows a shape as in Figure 7.3. At low quantities of medical personnel, the marginal effect would be very significant. From a certain quantity on, this marginal effect tapers off. An asymptotic level of life expectancy would be reached as soon as there is an abundance of medical personnel.

Non-linear cost functions
    One may have to estimate a *cost function* for, say, hospitals. Suppose we have cross-section data from a sample of hospitals. One may want to investigate whether hospitals generally display decreasing average costs up to a particular output level and

increasing average costs from that output level on.
The variable output may be approximated by the number
of patients, the number of hospital beds *etc*. Note
that decreasing costs may be obtained by the better
use of equipment and personnel as the hospital fa-
cility grows; increasing costs may be the result of
increasing management problems. The shape of the
curve corresponding to such a cost behavior is dis-
played in Figure 7.4.

Figure 7.4. Non-linear cost curve

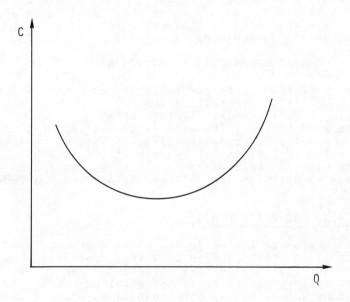

The appropriate specification is the following

$$C = \alpha + \beta Q + \gamma Q^2$$

where[15] C and Q refer to average cost and output,
respectively. The coefficients β and γ are expected
to be negative and positive, respectively.

7.4.2. DUMMY VARIABLES

Sometimes it is difficult to find a suitable measure
for an explanatory variable. Let us illustrate this
by means of the following example. Suppose we want

to estimate the relationship between the use of contraceptives and the literacy rate in developing countries by means of cross-section data. We would expect to find a positive relationship, in the sense that the more people are literate (and therefore educated), the more they are likely to understand the need for birth-control measures. We can reason, in addition, that people's religious feelings may also have a serious impact upon their choice regarding the use of contraceptives. Therefore, the hypothesis may be tested whether people in catholic LDC are more inhibited towards using contraceptives than people in non-catholic LDC. What to do about the variable 'faith' that seems so hard to quantify? The following equation is offered as a solution:

$$CONTRA = \alpha + \beta LIT + \gamma RELIGION$$

where CONTRA = percentage of married women using contraceptives
LIT = adult literacy rate.
The variable RELIGION will assume values of 1 if the country is predominantly catholic; it will have a value of 0 if it is predominantly non-catholic. The expected value of γ is negative. Variables such as RELIGION are referred to as *dummy* variables.

7.4.3. ECONOMETRIC MODELING

Many research topics do not require the study of merely one relationship between a dependent variable and a set of explanatory variables. Frequently the explanatory variables in one equation can be explained, in turn, by other equations. A set of equations that attempts to explain a series of interrelated phenomena is called a *model*. Econometric techniques such as RA are used to estimate the coefficients in a model's equations. An advantage of econometric modeling *vis-à-vis* the evaluation techniques discussed earlier is that it is more comprehensive and that explicit attention can be given to direct as well as indirect interactions between variables.

Let us next discuss the four types of equations in an econometric model[16]. First, *behavior* equations imply a number of assumptions about the economic behavior of individuals, the government, health personnel *etc*. For instance, the equation of the demand for health care by individuals is a

behavior equation, since it reveals how individuals'
health care demand changes as a result of movements
in variables such as price, income *etc.* Secondly,
technical equations usually describe the relation
between an output and a series of inputs. The notion
of output has to be understood in a wide sense here:
it not only refers to production of commodities or
services but it also encompasses output in terms of
life expectancy, lives saved due to health interventions, the birth rate, the weight and height of an
individual *etc.* The inputs are to be seen as technical determinants of the output. For instance,
the nutritional status may be considered as an input in the production of an individual's weight.
Thirdly, *institutional* equations reflect relationships imposed by law or custom. Suppose that in a
certain country, a complementarity is imposed between
the numbers of nurses and doctors. In that case,
regressing the variable 'nurses' on the variable
'doctors' would result in an institutional equation.
Fourthly, *identities* specify relations that are true
by definition. For instance, the variable 'population per doctor' is equal to the variable 'population' divided by the variable 'number of doctors'.

Variables are either *endogenous* or *predetermined*.
The former are always determined within the model.
The latter can be either lagged endogenous variables,
viz. variables whose values are determined in previous time periods within the model, or exogenous
variables that are determined outside the model.
The exogenous variables that are controlled by the
government can be called *policy* variables. For instance, a typical policy variable would be the government expenditures for the prevention of parasitic
diseases. If government has set certain *targets*
for the endogenous variables (*e.g.* life expectancy,
infant mortality, *etc.*), it will have to search for
the values of the policy variables that help to
satisfy these targets.

7.5. CASE STUDY: A MODEL OF THE LINKAGES BETWEEN HEALTH AND BASIC NEEDS

7.5.1. INTRODUCTION

As alluded to in the first chapter, the basic needs
approach to development became rather popular in the
mid-seventies. In this approach the fulfillment of
basic needs such as health, clothing, sanitation,

shelter, nutrition and education, is regarded upon as the key to rapid poverty eradication in LDC. A simple econometric model will now be constructed, using data of a sample of LDC on basic needs variables. The main purpose of this model is to show that there are important linkages between health and other basic needs variables[17]. The awareness of these linkages leads one to adopt a basic needs approach to health improvements. Economists involved in health planning should thus understand these linkages if they intend to design cost-effective health programs.

In the next section, we present the basic needs model. Information about the model's specification and data is given in 7.5.3. In section 7.5.4. an overview of the equations is presented. We comment upon the estimation results in 7.5.5. A conclusion is presented in 7.5.6.

7.5.2. A BASIC NEEDS MODEL

Health indicators
We start by explaining *life expectancy at birth in years*. This is widely accepted as one of the useful indicators of the health status of a population. It will be explained as follows:

$$LIFE_t = LIFE_t(PHY^+_{t-j}, NUR^+_{t-j}, CAL_{t-j}, AWS_{t-j}, LIT_{t-j}) (7.29)$$

where $LIFE$ = life expectancy at birth in years
PHY^+ = physicians per thousand population
NUR^+ = nurses per thousand population
CAL = daily calorie supply per capita as a percentage of requirement
AWS = percentage of population with access to safe water
LIT = adult literacy rate.

The subscripts in (7.29) refer to the time period; lagged variables occur whenever $j>0$. The first two explanatory variables in (7.29) refer to the *input of medical personnel*. The latter input is likely to have a beneficial impact upon health, hence it follows that the coefficients of PHY^+ and NUR^+ are expected to be positive. The variable CAL represents the *nutritional level* (in terms of calories) of the population. Low calorie levels will have a negative effect on LIFE due to a high death probability following malnutrition. Malnutrition may also diminish life expectancy in the sense that it reduces the

resistance to various infectious diseases. The effect of CAL on LIFE is therefore expected to be
positive. *Clean water supply* is also incorporated
in equation (7.29), in order to convey that availability of clean water may seriously diminish the
transmittal of dangerous parasitic and infectious
diseases; the effect of AWS on LIFE should therefore be positive. The effect of *literacy* on LIFE
is also presumed to be positive. The reasoning is
as follows. The literacy rate is a measure of the
degree of education of the population. The more
educated a population is, the better it understands
how the various health determinants can be manipulated in order to improve its health status. The
variable LIT therefore represents the intensity of
the utilization of PHY^*, NUR^*, CAL and AWS.

The other health indicators modeled are the
crude death rate and the child death rate:

$$CD_t = CD_t(PHY^*_{t-j}, NUR^*_{t-j}, AWS_{t-j}, CAL_{t-j}, LIT_{t-j}) \quad (7.30)$$

$$CRD_t = CRD_t(PHY^*_{t-j}, NUR^*_{t-j}, AWS_{t-j}, CAL_{t-j}, LIT_{t-j}) \quad (7.31)$$

CD and CRD refer to the child death rate among children (1-4 years old) and the crude death rate per
thousand population, respectively. One can see
that these equations feature the same determinants
as in the LIFE equation. The signs of the coefficients are expected to be opposite of those in the
LIFE equation, however.

Health determinants
We will first attempt to explain the health
determinants incorporated in equation (7.29). The
following type of function will be accepted:

$$Y_t = F(GNP_{t-j}) \quad (7.32)$$

where Y_t refers to a vector composed of PHY^*_t, NUR^*_t,
CAL_t, AWS_t and LIT_t; likewise, F is a vector of
functions. The variable GNP denotes as before the
per capita level of gross national product (in $).
GNP is further derived from the identity

$$GNP = TGNP/POP \quad (7.33),$$

where TGNP and POP refer to gross national product
and population, respectively.

GNP is a major explanatory variable in these

139

equations, in order to represent the idea that higher economic welfare can entail an improvement in basic needs. Indeed, the more developed a society becomes, the more it will be able to allocate funds to social services; it can, for instance, finance the education of additional doctors, nurses and midwives. Economic growth also facilitates improvements in the nutritional level of the population by means, for instance of higher investments in the agricultural sector. And as GNP rises, more resources can also be spent on clean water supply and basic education. We therefore consider growth of GNP to be potentially beneficial to the fulfillment of basic needs. The latter is also the view of Isenman(1980 ,p.246) who writes in an article about basic needs in Sri Lanka that 'the Sri Lankan experience sharply illustrates the commonsense point that without adequate growth countries will not have enough financial resources to maintain, let alone expand, basic-needs programmes'. *Population growth* exerts indirectly a negative influence upon the provision of basic needs. The reasoning is that, given a certain level of TGNP, the higher the population growth, the more difficult it becomes to provide a sufficient level of basic needs to every citizen.

Whereas TGNP will be kept exogenous in this study, further attention will be paid to the explanation of population growth. The following set of equations is therefore defined:

$$CRB_t = CRB_t(GNP_{t-j}, CD_{t-j}, CONTRA_{t-j}) \qquad (7.34)$$

$$CONTRA_t = CONTRA_t(PHY^+_{t-j}, NUR^+_{t-j}, LIT_{t-j}) \qquad (7.35)$$

$$POPGR_t = CRB_t - CRD_t \qquad (7.36)$$

$$POP_t = POP_{t-1}(1+POPGR_t) \qquad (7.37)$$

where CRB = crude birth rate per thousand population
      CONTRA = percentage of married women using
                  contraceptives
      POPGR = population growth.
The population growth rate in eq.(7.36) is equal to the birth rate minus the death rate. We will assume here that the importance of net immigration in explaining population is negligible. Hence this variable is omitted from eq.(7.36). In the *birth rate equation*, the level of GNP is expected to have a negative impact on CRB. GNP can be seen as a mea-

sure of the opportunity cost of having a child; the higher GNP (the higher therefore the opportunity cost), the more the demand for children will be de- pressed. The effect of the variable CONTRA in the birth rate equation should obviously be negative. The death rate among children, CD, is also considered to be an important determinant of CRB. Indeed, many parents in LDC try to compensate for the eventual loss of children by a high fertility rate. The main reason for this behavior is that in poor countries, where social security is usually non-existent, chil- dren are important because they contribute a lot to parents'economic security. *The use of contracep- tives by married women* is explained by the literacy rate. The literacy rate is presumed to have a pos- itive effect on the use of contraceptives, in the sense that it captures a better intellectual under- standing about the use and benefits of contraceptives. In other words it is likely to entail a higher effective use of contraceptives.

7.5.3. SPECIFICATION OF THE EQUATIONS AND THE DATA

Equations (7.29) to (7.31) can be described as tech- nical equations: they represent the impacts of health determinants in health inputs on health sta- tus. Eqs.(7.32), (7.34) and (7.35) are of the be- havioral type: eq.(7.32) conveys the behavior of governments with respect to basic needs as GNP rises whereas (7.34) and (7.35) reveal the behavior of families, concerning the demand for children and the use of contraceptives. Eqs.(7.33), (7.36) and (7.37) are identities.

The technical and behavior equations in the model are specified in a log-linear way[18]. This has the known advantage that estimated coefficients can be interpreted as elasticities[19]. Another fea- ture of the log-linear specification is that the marginal effects of explanatory variables decline as the values of the latter increase. The specified equations should be interpreted as valid in the short run only. Indeed, in the long run as LDC will become more and more developed, the dependent vari- ables in the model will tend to certain asymptotic values. The latter phenomenon would require another specification.

In the case of PHY$^+$ and NUR$^+$, GNP deliberately enters the equations with a lag of seven and three years, respectively, in order to convey that it takes an appropriate number of years before additional doctors and nurses are graduated. GNP with a one year lag is used in the equations of ASW, CAL and LIT so as to indicate that it takes at least one year before an increased allocation of funds towards these basic needs result in an actual improvement. In the other equations, the choice of the lags are mainly dictated by data availability. To give the reader more precise information about the years associated with the data and the time lags involved, an overview of the model is given in the next section.

Concerning the cross-section estimation of the model, we have relied on country data for LDC provided in the World Development Reports of the World Bank (1978, 1979, 1980b, 1981, 1982), the World Bank Atlas of 1977 and the Yearbook of National Accounts Statistics of the United Nations (1980). For the list of countries that constitute the sample, see Appendix 5.

7.5.4. OVERVIEW OF THE MODEL TO BE ESTIMATED[20]

$$life_t = a_0 + b_0 phy^*_{t-3} + c_0 nur^*_{t-3} + d_0 cal_{t-3} + e_0 asw_{t-5} + f_0 lit_{t-3} \quad (t=1980)$$

$$phy^*_t = a_1 + b_1 gnp_{t-7} \quad (t=1977)$$

$$nur^*_t = a_2 + b_2 gnp_{t-3} \quad (t=1977)$$

$$cal_t = a_3 + b_3 gnp_{t-1} \quad (t=1977)$$

$$asw_t = a_4 + b_4 gnp_{t-1} \quad (t=1975)$$

$$lit_t = a_5 + b_5 gnp_{t-1} \quad (t=1977)$$

$$crb_t = a_6 + b_6 gnp_{t-1} + c_6 contra_{t-2} + d_6 cd_{t-2} \quad (t=1980)$$

$$contra_t = a_7 + b_7 lit_{t-1} \quad (t=1978)$$

$$cd_t = a_8 + b_8 phy^*_{t-3} + c_8 nur^*_{t-3} + d_8 cal_{t-3} + e_8 asw_{t-5} + f_8 lit_{t-3} \quad (t=1980)$$

$$crd_t = a_9 + b_9 phy^*_{t-3} + c_9 nur^*_{t-3} + d_9 cal_{t-3} + e_9 asw_{t-5} + f_9 lit_{t-3} \quad (t=1980)$$

$$POPGR_t = CRB_t - CRD_t$$

$$POP_t = POP_{t-1}(1 + POPGR_t)$$

$$GNP_t = TGNP_t / POP_t$$

7.5.5. ESTIMATION RESULTS

The model is estimated by means of RA. The results are presented in Table 7.3. All coefficients appear to have the correct sign. It can also be verified that, in quite a number of cases, the coefficients are statistically different from zero at the 5 per cent or 10 per cent significance level. The estimates clearly show that linkages between health status and basic needs variables exist. These linkages are portrayed in Figure 7.5. The model therefore strongly suggests that a health program based on the basic needs idea is an economically efficient way of attacking poor health.

GNP is also an important variable in the equations explaining the basic needs levels. This shows that economic growth can contribute to the provision of basic needs. More precisely, GNP can be understood in this model as a variable that *finances* improvements of basic needs. Let us make a further assessment now of certain coefficient estimates. *First*, the coefficients of health personnel in the health status equations reveal that they are most efficient in combatting child death. *Secondly*, the calorie-elasticity in the child death equation is remarkably high, demonstrating that nutrition intervention policies will be very effective in reducing excessive child death. *Thirdly*, literacy seems to be an important health determinant as well as the major variable explaining the use of contraceptives. Education programs constitute therefore another efficient way of achieving, directly or indirectly, a better health.

It is evident that the model intends to capture the major determinants of poor health only. Variables that are country-specific such as government health policies (*e.g.* food subsidies, adequate network of rural hospitals, special measures against tropical diseases, *etc.*) are not represented in the model; that is why in some equations the $\bar{R}^2$ remains rather low, of course.

7.5.6. CONCLUSION

The estimates show that linkages between health and various basic needs variables definitely exist. They thus show that health has a wide range of direct and indirect determinants. Hence, health planners ought

Table 7.3. Coefficient estimates of the basic needs model

Table 7.3 on p. 144 should read as follows:

Dependent variables	Explanatory variables									$\bar{R}^2$	Standard error of estimate
	constant	phy*	nur*	cal	asw	lit	gnp	contra	cd		
life	3.0819 (0.5565)	0.0484 (0.0153)	0.0122 (0.0152)	0.1151 (0.1222)	0.0271 (0.0209)	0.0991 (0.0207)				0.7795	C.078
phy*	-8.9480 (0.7893)						1.3456 (0.1528)			0.6048	0.7576
nur*	-4.8349 (0.7249)						0.7215 (0.1296)			0.3749	0.6998
cal	4.0824 (0.1049)						0.0859 (0.0181)			0.3015	0.0980
asw	-0.4012 (0.5784)						0.6699 (0.1034)			0.4503	0.5583
lit	0.3116 (0.6584)						0.5773 (0.1134)			0.3325	0.6149
crb	3.4757 (0.3446)						-0.0034 (.0460)	-0.0505 (0.0429)	0.1134 (0.0599)	0.4751	0.1266
contra	-3.6019 (0.7914)					1.6270 (0.1989)				0.7762	0.5235
cd	9.8393 (4.1850)	-0.2276 (0.1149)	-0.0619 (0.1144)	-1.2791 (0.9191)	-0.0023 (0.1570)	-0.5015 (0.1555)				0.5868	0.5899
crd	6.0075 (1.5980)	-0.1034 (0.0439)	-0.0596 (0.0437)	-0.6047 (0.3510)	-0.0187 (0.0599)	-0.2213 (0.0594)				0.7000	0.2253

Note: - Figures between brackets refer to standard errors of coefficients.
 - In the case of the equations for crb and contra, the observations amounted to twenty (for the countries included in this sample, see Appendix 5). The latter is due to the lack of data on CONTRA. For the other equations, the sample consisted of 51 observations.

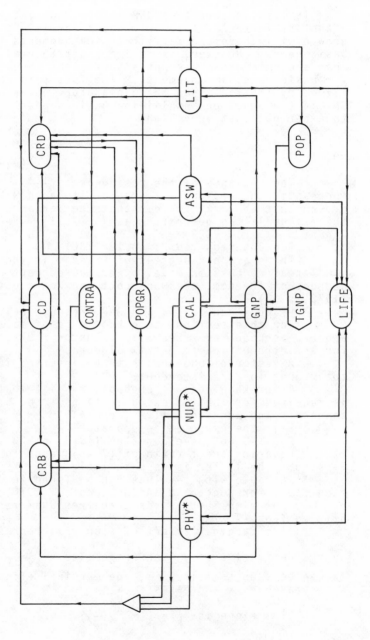

Figure 7.5. Linkages between basic needs variables

to take notice of these determinants if they want to design cost-effective health programs.

It is also seen that GNP is an important explanatory factor of the basic needs levels. Economic growth will therefore facilitate improvements in basic needs. However, it is important to realize that economic growth is not a sufficient condition for basic needs improvements. The latter is confirmed by the fact that the explanatory power of GNP in the equations explaining basic needs is altogether not that very high.

NOTES

[1] The variance of the residuals is $\dfrac{\sum\limits_{i=1}^{n} (e_i - \bar{e})^2}{n}$, where $\bar{e}$ is the residuals' average. It can now be proven that $\bar{e}=0$. It follows that the variance of the residuals can be written as in (7.11). See also Johnston (1972, p.129).

[2] See Johnston (1972, pp.128-130).

[3] There are $n-2$ degrees of freedom in the simple linear regression model. For the concept of degrees of freedom, see Wonnacott and Wonnacott (1970, p.52).

[4] y and x denote EXP and GNP, respectively.

[5] For this section, some knowledge of matrix algebra is required. See *e.g.* Johnston (1972, ch.4) for an introduction to matrix algebra.

[6] A vector of ones needs to be inserted in X to account for the intercept.

[7] Prior knowledge of probability distributions is required for the following sections. See *e.g.* Wonnacott and Wonnacott (1970, ch.14).

[8] E is the expectation operator.

[9] For a proof, see Johnston (1972, p.128).

[10] Squaring the t-ratio of (7.26) leads to a F-ratio. The latter is used in Table 1.9.

[11] A table with t-values can be found in Johnston (1972) or Wonnacott and Wonnacott (1970).

[12] For simplicity's sake, the residual term is omitted from (7.27).

[13] The marginal effect of x on y is represented by the derivative of y with respect to x: $\dfrac{\partial y}{\partial x} = \beta_1 \beta_2 x^{\beta_2 - 1}$. It can be seen that if $\beta_2 < 1$, the marginal effect of x decreases as x increases.

[14] The slope is $\dfrac{\partial y}{\partial x} = e^{\alpha - \frac{\beta}{x}} \left(\dfrac{\beta}{x^2}\right)$.

146

[15] The slope of this function is $\frac{\partial C}{\partial Q} = \beta + 2\gamma Q$.

[16] See Barten (1981).

[17] For a similar study, see Wheeler (1980). There are a few differences between his and our model, however. Namely, we introduce more health variables and more linkages between the basic needs variables. In our model, we do not attempt to explain the growth of the national product, however.

[18] This is equivalent to a double-log transformation.

[19] We refer to section 7.4.1. We derive from equation (7.28) that the derivative of ln y with respect to ln x, $\frac{\partial \ln y}{\partial \ln x}$, is equal to β_2. We can also write that $\frac{\partial \ln y}{\partial \ln x} = \frac{\Delta y/y}{\Delta x/x}$, where Δ denotes a 'small variation'. It follows that β_2 can be interpreted as the percentage change of y caused by a change of x by one per cent. The coefficient β_2 is also called *elasticity*.

[20] Symbols written in lowercase refer to logarithmic transformation of the original variables. The time period to which the data pertain is only given for the equations to be estimated, of course.

Chapter Eight

POLICY EVALUATION BY SIMULATION

8.1. DEFINITION

We know that an econometric model gives information
about the relationships between endogenous and explanatory variables. Policy evaluation consists of
studying the effects of alternative policies on *target* variables. The latter are endogenous variables
that are of special interest to the policy-makers.
Note that policy evaluation is one of the principal
aims of model construction. It is generally carried
out by means of computer simulation. Below, we will
outline this technique by using the basic needs model presented in the previous chapter.

8.2. CALCULATION OF POLICY RESPONSES

8.2.1. INTRODUCTION

Policy-makers mainly evaluate policies by means of
policy responses. Such responses are the effects
of a change in policy on the chosen target variables.
Before they can be calculated, a *base case* simulation has to be carried out: it is essentially a *projection* by means of the model, thereby assuming that
the exogenous variables follow a *normal* course. In
other words, in a base case simulation no special
policy alternative is to be used. Once the base case simulation is ready, *policy simulations* can be
performed. The latter are obtained as a result of
introducing alternative sets of values for the policy variables. A set of such values constitutes a *policy*. The policy responses corresponding to a particular policy are estimated by the differences between
the values of the target variables in the policy
and in the base case simulation[1].

8.2.2. COMPUTER SIMULATION WITH A RECURSIVE MODEL

Models that are *recursive* are fairly simple to work
with. Recursiveness means that a model's equations
can be arranged in such a way that each equation,
having endogenous variables among the explanatory
variables, only features endogenous variables that
are explained by equations ranked earlier in the model. The solution of a recursive model is easy:
starting the simulation in a particular year with
a given set of values for the exogenous and lagged
endogenous variables, the whole model can be solved,
for each year considered, in one single iteration.

Many models are not recursive, however. They
frequently contain endogenous variables that are,in
turn, explained by other endogenous variables *in
the same time period*. This makes it necessary to
use iterative solution techniques such as the Gauss-
Seidel method[2]. In this chapter, we will restrict
ourselves to the computer simulation of recursive
models, however.

8.3. SETTING UP A SIMULATION EXPERIMENT WITH THE BASIC NEEDS MODEL

8.3.1. THE BASIC NEEDS MODEL AS A RECURSIVE MODEL

The basic needs model[3] of the previous chapter happens to be recursive. A ranking of the equations
confirming the recursive nature of the model is
given in Table 8.1. We will show briefly why this
model is easy to solve.

Table 8.1. Ranking of equations of the basic needs
model for recursiveness

Number of ranking	Endogenous variable
1	CRB
2	CRD
3	POPGR
4	POP
5	GNP
6	PHY*
7	NUR*
8	CAL
9	ASW
10	LIT

Table 8.1. (cont'd')

Number of ranking	Endogenous variable
11	CONTRA
12	CD
13	LIFE

Suppose we want to compute a base case solution, starting in the year 1980 and ending in 1995. Given the value of GNP for 1979, the value of CD and CONTRA for 1978, CRB for 1980 can readily be calculated. Subsequently, given the values of PHY^*, NUR^*, CAL, ASW and LIT for the appropriate years before 1980, CRD can be computed. Population growth, POPGR, in 1980 can be derived from the previously found values for CRB and CRD. Given POPGR for 1980 and total population in 1979, the total population, POP, in 1980 can be calculated. Gross national product per capita, GNP, is then derived from TGNP, that is exogenous, and POP. The equations for the remaining endogenous variables only need exogenous variables and lagged values of endogenous variables; hence they can be solved without any problem. This will complete the solution of the model for the year 1980. For the subsequent years, it suffices to repeat the above procedure. In the next section, we will discuss the steps of a simulation experiment in greater detail.

8.3.2. A DIGRESSION ON THE STEPS OF A SIMULATION EXPERIMENT

We assume that the estimated basic needs model can be applied to any developing country that is part of our sample. In other words, for each projection pertaining to a different country, we will accept the same set of coefficient estimates. Once we have selected the country for our simulation experiment, the following steps have to be taken:
Step 1
First, one has to make a decision about whether or not we will *calibrate* the equations to the observations of the base or starting year of the simulation. In our experiments, 1980 will be designed as the base year. Calibration means that, given the appropriate set of exogenous and lagged endogenous vari-

ables, the constant term in each equation is adjusted in such a way that the observed values of the endogenous variables in the base year can be reproduced without error.

Earlier we said that the equations do not contain all possible explanatory variables; indeed, we only focused on the main determinants of health status and basic needs. A disadvantage of such an approach is, that the explanatory power of the regressions is sometimes rather low. Thus, if we were to use the estimated equations directly in the simulation experiment, we would seriously underestimate or overestimate the true values of a number of endogenous variables. It is clear that we can somehow take account of this problem by calibrating the equations: it implies an upward or downward adjustment of the estimated constant term. We may view this adjustment as the influence of all explanatory variables that are omitted from the model. This adjustment is sometimes referred to as an *add factor*[4]. Note that in the simulation exercises to be discussed, we have opted for the calibration of the equations.

Step 2
One writes a computer program in which the calibrated equations appear in a recursive way.

Step 3
Values (from 1973 to 1979) for TGNP, population and the lagged endogenous variables, that appear as explanatory variables in the equations, are to be fed into the computer program. We need values from 1973 on, due to the presence of a seven year-lag in the model. Wherever it is feasible, data are taken from published sources. If data for certain years are not available, reasonable assumptions about them will have to be made. Sometimes we let the variable assume a value that is equal to that of the closest observation. In other cases, values are derived from the application of a growth rate to observations that are close in time.

Step 4
We project of a likely course for TGNP for the length of the simulation period adopted, namely from 1980 to 1995[5].

Step 5
We now make a projection, from 1980 to 1995, of all

151

endogenous variables. Note that since we have calibrated the equations to the base year data, the
'projected' values for 1980 will be identical to
the observations of 1980. Eventually during the
course of the projection, the model will have to
use the lagged endogenous variables as they are
computed in the simulation. In other words, there
are linkages between simulated variables of different
time periods: one therefore speaks of a *dynamic* type
of simulation.

Step 6
We save the base case simulation as a benchmark for
comparison with the policy simulations.

Step 7
We define a policy alternative or *scenario*. It consists of an alternative course for the policy variables *from 1980 on*. Furthermore, we adopt the same
set of values for the TGNP, population and lagged
endogenous variables, from 1973 to 1979, as in Step
3. Given this information, we are able to perform
a policy simulation. It is evident that we can repeat the present step whenever we are interested in
a new scenario.

It is true that TGNP clearly manifests itself
in the model as the only policy variable[6]. However,
in our simulation exercise we can also apply the add
factor technique. In a policy simulation, an add
factor can be added to an equation's intercept by
the policy-maker so as to represent policy changes
that cannot be captured by changes in TGNP. For
instance, a massive investment in clear water supply
can hardly be represented adequately by a change in
TGNP. Hence, the possibility exists to adjust the
intercept in the ASW equation upwards so as to convey the implementation of a policy geared especially
to the development of clean water distribution.
Hence, a scenario consists of perturbations in GNP,
the use of add factors or a combination of both.

Step 8
By deducting the values of the endogenous variables
obtained from the base case simulation from those
of the policy simulations, we obtain the policy
responses of each scenario.

Step 9
The final step for the policy-maker is to select the
best strategy out of the set of simulated scenarios.

If there is but one target variable, the selection
is easy: one merely adopts the scenario that comes
as near to the target as possible. If there are
many target variables, it becomes appropriate to
use multiattribute problem analysis. The policy
responses constitute an ideal framework for checking
which policy alternatives are most efficient in
reaching predetermined targets.

8.4. CASE STUDY: A SIMULATION EXPERIMENT WITH THE
BASIC NEEDS MODEL APPLIED TO RWANDA

8.4.1. INTRODUCTION

First we gather the data necessary to compute the
calibrated constants and to start the simulation.
These are given in Table 8.2. The calibrated constants themselves are listed in Table 8.3. The figures used are based upon the data for Rwanda listed
in the World Development Report of the World Bank
(1982). One can see that in a number of cases the
values are kept constant through time. Note also
that GNP is expressed in dollars of 1980.

In the base case solution, we assume that the
total gross national product (TGNP) of Rwanda grows,
in real terms, by 4.6 per cent. The scenarios are
the following:

Scenario 1: TGNP grows by 5.6 per cent

Scenario 2: LIT is augmented yearly by 10 units via
an add factor[7]

Scenario 3: CAL is augmented yearly by 10 units by
means of an add factor[8]

Scenario 4: PHY* is augmented yearly (taking account
of a seven year-lag, however) by 0.02
units by means of an add factor[9]

Scenario 5: Add factors[10] are used such that LIT
and CAL are augmented by 3 units and
PHY* by 0.01.

Table 8.2. Values used to start the simulation experiments and to calibrate the equations to the data of 1980

Variables	Years							
	1973	1974	1975	1976	1977	1978	1979	1980
CRB								53
CRD								20
POP							5,033,880	5,200,000
GNP	182.711	185.086	187.492	189.930	192.399	194.900	197.433	200
PHY[+]					0.02577	0.02577	0.02577	0.02577
NUR[+]					0.0956	0.0956	0.0956	0.0956
CAL					94	94	94	94
ASW			35	35	35	35	35	35
LIT					50	50	50	50
CONTRA						5	5	5
CD						27	27	27
LIFE								45

Table 8.3. Calibrated constants

Equation	Calibrated constants
CRB	3.6958
CRD	6.1571
PHY*	-10.6663
NUR*	-6.1423
CAL	4.0893
ASW	0.0147
LIT	0.8608
CONTRA	-4.7554
CD	10.0992
LIFE	3.0054

8.4.2. POLICY RESPONSES

In Table 8.4, we present the base case solution together with the policy responses of the five scenarios. Remember that we define a policy response
as being equal to the simulation minus the base case
value. The results will only be given for a number
of selected years.

A few comments are in order about the most important policy responses in the different scenarios.
It can be seen that a *growth* scenario (scenario 1)
results in a number of improvements: the values of
all basic needs variables increase, leading to a
better health status that is represented by a lower
child and crude death rate and by a higher life expectancy. Population hardly changes *vis-à-vis* the
base case value. The *literacy* scenario (scenario 2)
has a fairly large effect upon the crude birth rate.
The latter is the result of a greater use of contraceptives and a lower child death rate, generated by
the increase in literacy. Population decreases, compared to the base case, which entails a somewhat
higher GNP and higher values for the basic needs
variables. The *calorie* scenario (scenario 3) illustrates that child death is particularly sensitive
to calorie intake. Total population increases such
that GNP decreases. The latter entails a small
decrease in the levels of a number of basic needs
variables. The *physicians* scenario (scenario 4) is
similar to the previous one: it shows a significant
effect on child mortality, whereas the basic needs
variables, apart from PHY*, decrease due to a lower
GNP. The latter is caused by the rise in population.

The last scenario is a *combination* of exogenous increases in LIT, CAL and PHY*. Therefore, the policy responses obtained are similar to those of scenarios 2 to 4.

The simulation experiment confirms an important characteristic of the basic needs model, namely that the provision of basic needs can be enhanced and a better health status can be obtained by means of a higher economic growth. In other words, according to the model, a growth policy seems to be as good as a more direct basic needs policy. As we discussed in chapters 1 and 2, this is not necessarily the case in reality, however. Let us reiterate our opinion on this matter: a growth policy is, implicitly, equivalent to a basic needs policy, only if a suffi- cient part of the additional resources, that are made available by higher growth, are directed towards a better provision of basic needs!

8.4.3. THE CHOICE OF AN OPTIMAL STRATEGY

The selection of a best strategy depends on the pre- ferences of the policy-makers, of course. If life expectancy is the only target variable, for instance, the fourth scenario should be chosen. Scenario 3 should be selected if the child death rate is to be minimized. If the minimization of the child death rate and a maximization of life expectancy are the policy-makers' objectives, one is confronted with a multiattribute problem: indeed, scenarios 3 to 5 prove to be non-dominated alternatives. It follows that policy-makers ought to formulate their value judgments about the relative importance of child death and life expectancy in order to select an op- timal strategy.

The present simulation experiment has shown that an econometric model can be a useful tool in decision-making. The construction of models of entire health systems should, therefore, definitely be encouraged.

Table 8.4. Base case values and policy responses for selected years

Endogenous variables	Base case values	Policy responses				
		Scenario 1	Scenario 2	Scenario 3	Scenario 4	Scenario 5
Crude birth rate (‰) (CRB)						
1980	53.00	0	0	0	0	0
1985	52.92	-0.0307	-1.3144	-0.7700	0	-0.6620
1990	52.47	-0.2525	-1.2639	-0.7464	0	-0.6377
1995	52.03	-0.5505	-1.2247	-0.7243	-0.6656	-0.9889
Crude death rate (‰) (CRD)						
1980	20.00	0	0	0	0	0
1985	19.81	-0.0339	-0.7734	-1.1727	0	-0.6177
1990	19.35	-0.2379	-0.7343	-1.1276	-1.0189	-1.1547
1995	18.91	-0.5622	-0.7063	-1.0819	-0.9273	-1.0770
Population growth (%) (POPGR)						
1980	3.30	0	0	0	0	0
1985	3.31	0.0003	-0.0541	0.0403	0	-0.0044
1990	3.31	-0.0014	-0.0530	0.0381	0.1019	0.0517
1995	3.31	0.0012	-0.0518	0.0358	0.0262	0.0088

Table 8.4. (cont'd')

Endogenous variables	Base case values	Policy responses					
		Scenario 1	Scenario 2	Scenario 3	Scenario 4	Scenario 5
Population (POP)						
1980	5,200,000	0	0	0	0	0
1985	6,117,400	-42.5	-3,187	16,406	0	4,158
1990	7,199,680	-61.5	-18,063	32,903	7,100	7,208
1995	8,473,650	446.0	-47,668	53,862	25,534	15,764
Gross National Product per capita (GNP)						
1980	200.00	0	0	0	0	0
1985	212.88	0.9430	0	-0.0559	0	-0.0177
1990	226.48	2.2467	0.0662	-0.1067	0	-0.0128
1995	240.96	3.7012	0.1368	-0.1589	-0.0731	-0.0471
Number of physicians per thousand population (PHY)						
1980	0.0258	0	0	0	0	0
1985	0.0281	0	0	0	0	0
1990	0.0306	0.0012	0	0	0.02	0.0099
1995	0.0333	0.0036	0.0001	-0.0002	0.02	0.0099

Number of nurses per
thousand population
(NUR•)

Year						
1980	0.0956	0	0	0	0	0
1985	0.1001	0.0014	0.0001	0	0	0
1990	0.1047	0.0052	0.0001	-0.0003	0	0
1995	0.1095	0.0094	0.0003	-0.0004	-0.0002	-0.0001

Calorie intake per
capita as percentage
of requirement
(CAL)

Year						
1980	94.00	0	0	10	0	3
1985	94.51	0.3096	0	9.9814	0	2.9942
1990	95.01	0.7014	0.0212	9.9658	0	2.9959
1995	95.52	1.0989	0.0422	-9.9509	-0.0226	2.9855

Percentage of popu-
lation with access
to safe water
(ASW)

Year						
1980	35.00	0	0	0	0	0
1985	36.51	0.9430	0	-0.0559	0	-0.0177
1990	38.05	2.2467	0.0662	-0.1067	0	-0.0128
1995	39.67	3.7012	0.1368	-0.1589	-0.0731	-0.0471

Adult literacy rate
(LIT)

Year						
1980	50.00	0	10	0	0	3
1985	51.85	1.1521	10	-0.0685	0	2.9784
1990	53.74	2.7232	10.0800	-0.1298	0	2.9845
1995	55.69	4.4505	10.1655	-0.1923	-0.0885	2.9430

Table 8.4. (Cont'd')

Endogenous variables	Base case values	Policy responses				
		Scenario 1	Scenario 2	Scenario 3	Scenario 4	Scenario 5
Use of contraceptives (as a percentage of married women) (CONTRA)						
1980	5.00	0	0	0	0	0
1985	5.24	0.1425	1.7556	-0.0056	0	0.5043
1990	5.56	0.4118	1.8041	-0.0199	0	0.5143
1995	5.84	0.7255	1.8577	-0.0311	-0.0318	0.5191
Child death rate (%$_o$) (CD)						
1980	27.00	0	0	0	0	0
1985	26.49	-0.1005	-2.2848	-3.2065	0	-1.7636
1990	25.26	-0.6127	-2.1197	-3.0142	-2.8346	-3.1818
1995	24.10	-1.4112	-1.9869	-2.8282	-2.5254	-2.9019
Life expectancy at birth in years (LIFE)						
1980	45.00	0	0	0	0	0
1985	45.16	0.0288	0.8123	0.5275	0	0.4220
1990	45.62	0.2221	0.7966	0.5179	1.1697	1.0764
1995	46.07	0.5763	0.7903	0.5041	1.0990	1.0261

NOTES

[1] If the model is linear, the policy responses to a small change in policy variables can also be derived from the matrix of coefficient estimates. See *e.g.* Intriligator (1971, ch.16).
[2] See Naylor (1971) or Barten (1981).
[3] The reader is strongly advised to come to grips with the mechanism of the model as presented in chapter 7, before continuing the study of the present chapter.
[4] See Intriligator (1971, p.516-517).
[5] We consider this period to be a 'short' period in the history of economic development of a developing country.
[6] It is thus assumed here that the policy-maker can manipulate gross national product.
[7] This corresponds to adding 2.302585 to the calibrated constant.
[8] *Ibidem.*
[9] The add factor amounts to -3.912023.
[10] The add factor used in the equations for LIT and CAL is 1.098612 whereas it is -4.605170 in the equation for PHY*.

Chapter Nine

HEALTH PLANNING

9.1. DEFINITION

Sorkin (1976, p.79) states that health planning 'involves the utilization of a series of analytic prag-
matic techniques to rationally allocate health resources for a specific period of time, usually rang-
ing from 1 to 10 years'. Health planning is, therefore, to be understood as an instrument that can be
used to improve a population's health status. In
this chapter, we will describe the planning process
as outlined by the WHO[1]. *Country Health Programming*,
as the WHO calls its planning approach is a 'process
designed to identify priority health problems of
prime concern to countries in this context of their
development plan; to specify targets in these problem areas, to translate targets into health development programmes, to be accomplished during a plan
period, through the identification of activities,
resource needs and organization required to attain
these objectives; and to implement, evaluate and
reformulate such programmes on a continuing basis'[2].
Note that this particular approach stresses the interaction between the health sector and other socio-
economic sectors of the economy.

9.2. COUNTRY HEALTH PROGRAMMING[3] (CHP)

9.2.1. INTRODUCTION

The preparation of the program proposals, supervising evaluating and reformulating them, when required,
is the responsibility of a group of high-ranking
officials and of experts. Henceforth, the latter
will be referred to as the GHP Group. The WHO re-
commends the following composition for this Group:

a top-ranking public health administrator, a senior
non-medical Health Administrator, a member of the
Planning Commission, a management expert, a health
economist, a statistician-demographer, an epidemi-
ologist, a social scientist and a representative of
the users of health services. Governments may ask
the WHO to help them implementing CHP. Note that
CHP was first introduced in Bangladesh in 1973.
Subsequently, from 1973 to 1977, 23 countries started CHP, whereas in 1977/1978, 12 countries showed
an interest in applying CHP.

9.2.2. A SUMMARY OF STAGES AND STEPS IN CHP

STAGE 1. Data collection, analysis and presentation

Step 1. Data collection

The data are to be collected at low cost; data that
are already available and are suitable, should be
used by the CHP Group. The data needed include the
following:

Demographic data and forecasts
        The aim of collecting demographic data is to
arrive at population forecasts that are to be used
when setting health targets and developing health
strategies. The data required consist of the age-
structure of the population, sex and marital composition, rural/urban distribution, birth rates, infant mortality and crude death rates.

Economic data
        A forecast of the gross domestic or gross na-
tional products is a minimum requirement. Government
revenues and expenditures are also of interest to
the CHP Group. These economic data can be used in
estimating the constraints of the growth of the national health budget and in assessing the impact of
development policy in general on the health sector.

Health status data
        Data on the disease situation will be of help
in setting health priorities and defining targets
for the program period. By disease situation, one
understands information on the mortality and morbidity rates (by age, sex and location if possible) by
disease groups.

Health and environmental health services
This type of information relates to the availability of health establishments, health manpower
and environmental health services. In addition, it
should be estimated how much of the population is
covered by these services in rural and urban areas.

Unit cost data
Concerning the existing service programs, information is needed about the cost per unit of activity (*i.e.* cost per vaccination, cost for case
finding, cost for a hospital bed/day, cost for a
health clinic visit *etc.*). The components of these
costs (*i.e.* salaries, maintenance and other recur-
ring costs, materials and equipment, transportation
etc.) should also be analyzed.

Policy data
The CHP Group should collect information about
policy data on national development policy, goals
and objectives and on national health policy.

Step 2. Data analysis and presentation

Once the data are collected, an information document
should be written about the health situation and,
wherever it is appropriate, the general development
in the country. The document has to be readable
and should not be restricted to a sheer listing of
statistical tables.

STAGE 2. Situation analysis and preperation of
program proposals

Step 3. Review of information document

The CHP Group has to review and, wherever needed,
rewrite the information document. It should also
be verified whether the data used are accurate and
whether the document describes the current situation
in the economy and in the health sector accurately.

Step 4. Problem definition

Health and health-related problems have now to be
identified by the CHP Group. There may be disease-
oriented problems, problems in the provision of
health services and the availability of health man-

power, and, finally, environmental health deficiencies. The list of problems should also include the effects of diseases upon economic development in general.

Step 5. Identification of problem/output indicators

One should attempt at constructing indices that measure changes in health and health-related problems. They are to be based on the collected data. If such indices prove to be difficult to produce, outputs of health activities can be used as an index.

Step 6. Identification of current activities addressed to health and health-related problems

For each problem, a list should be made, containing the health activities that are directed towards the disappearance of the problem.

Step 7. Identification of current resource allocation

Here, the CHP Group has to identify the resources that are currently used in the health activities initiated to solve the various health problems.

Step 8. Target setting

For a number of problems, it is likely that national health plans have defined already corresponding targets. The CHP Group will have to formulate its own targets for the problems not treated in those plans. It has to be checked carefully whether the targets are realistic and/or whether they can be adjusted up or downwards. Account has to be taken, here,of available resources in the present and in the future. Note that the targets for all problems must be related to the same period.

Step 9. Definition of health strategies

A *health strategy* can be defined as a group of interrelated medical, public health and health-related

techniques that can be organized to achieve a certain target. The CHP group has to work out, as
much as possible, alternative health strategies
that can meet the same target. Note that the quantity of the resources involved is not yet to be
specified here.

Step 10. Constraints analysis of strategies

It has to be verified whether the health strategies
can be organized, managed and applied in the social,
cultural, religious and political climate of the
country. If such constraints exist, it should be
investigated whether and how they can be overcome
in the future.

Step 11. Translation of strategies into health
         development programs

The health strategies that are not subject to the
constraints mentioned above, or for which the constraints have been eliminated, have to be transformed into *health development programs*. A health
development program defines which physical, human
and financial resources and institutional changes
are needed for the implementation of a strategy
aimed at a certain target. It gives more detailed
information about the techniques and procedures
that will be adopted. In addition, the program
specifies the target population, the institutional
and political changes required, if necessary, and
the resources needed to implement it. For each
health development program, the CHP group has to
estimate the cost of manpower, constructions, equipment, supplies, logistic support and information
services. A time-table has also to be set up for
each program.

Step 12. Constraints analysis of health development
         programs

First, the CHP Group must be concerned with the
support requirements for each program. This means
that it has to be investigated 'how manpower, manpower training, construction, logistics, supplies
and equipment, management and an adequate information
flow can be provided at the right place and time
during the implementation of the proposed health

development programme'⁴. For those programs that
appear not to be feasible, the reasons why have to
be stated together with an assessment of whether
the requirements can be met at some later time.
For implementable programs, the CHP Group has to
remain concerned with the most efficient use of the
scarce resources.

Secondly, it must be analyzed whether the alternative health development programs are *cost-
effective*. In other words, the Group has to check
whether low cost technologies are selected for
reaching the targets set forth in the development
programs. Subsequently, it has to be studied in
which way the programs will be *financed, i.e.* either
from the public sector, the private sector, social
security institutions or external agencies. The
latter analysis will indicate which programs are
not financially feasible. For the non-implementable
programs, one has to state the causes together with
the likelihood of implementation in the future.

Thirdly, the social and economic repercussions
of the programs have to be investigated. In other
words, each program's positive and adverse effects
on national objectives have to be analyzed.

After going through the three constraints analyses, it should be clear which programs are uncon-
ditionally feasible. One is then ready for the
preparation of the CHP document.

Step 13. Preparation of the CHP document

This document consists mainly of a description of
the procedures in stages 1 and 2, and of the health
development programs that are implementable as well
as non-implementable.

Step 14. Submission of the CHP document

The document has to be submitted to the Minister
of Health.

STAGE 3. Decision on program proposals

The government has to decide which of the alternative
health development programs have to be implemented.

STAGE 4. Continuation and integration of CHP in country's health structure

Steps 15 and 16. Project formulation and implementation

The formulation and implementation of projects may follow upon the acceptance of specific health development programs. The WHO defines a health project as a *temporary* intensive effort aimed at reducing a specific health or health-related problem. Examples of projects are a training program for village health workers, the construction of toilets, the initiation of a TBC control program *etc*. It is evident that a health development program may result in several health projects. The management of health projects in itself is not an easy matter. Readers that are interested in that aspect of health planning are referred to Bainbridge and Sapirie (1974).

9.2.3. CHP IN SRI LANKA

To illustrate the main features of CHP, we will present a brief discussion of CHP in Sri Lanka[5]. CHP was initiated in Sri Lanka in 1978. Sri Lanka had already an important health sector that was mainly directed towards curative medicine. CHP has changed this orientation by emphasizing preventive medicine and public health. *Eleven critical areas* were identified:

(i) Provision of safe and adequate water

It was recognized that clear water is essential for good health. Sri Lanka, having an access to safe water of 15 per cent, aimed at a water supply coverage of 50 per cent within the first 5 years of the CHP.

(ii) Sewage disposal and the provision of sanitary latrines

In rural and urban areas, the coverage in 1978 of sewage disposal and latrines was 50 and 60 per cent, respectively. The target in the 1978 health plan was to provide a coverage of 100 per cent within 5 years.

168

(iii) Health education

Again the target was a 100 per cent coverage within a period of 5 years. Health education included nutrition education, family health education, malaria and education of children on personal hygiene, use of water, latrines, dangers of smoking and the proper use of roads to limit accidents.

(iv) Immunization of newborns and infants

The target was to administer to 80-100 per cent of newborns and infants a BCG and DPT vaccine, respectively.

(v) Immunization of dogs

One aimed at a vaccination (against rabies) of all dogs within a period of 5 years.

(vi) Spraying in malaria infected areas

Prior to CHP, the coverage of malaria spraying was 70 per cent. In order to reduce the risk of death due to malaria, the target was to spray insecticides in all infected areas within 5 years.

(vii) Family planning services

Family planning was practised by only 19 per cent of the population in 1977. In order to achieve a stable population of 15 million, the aim was to introduce family planning in all families within 5 years.

(viii) Disposal of refuse and fly control measures

It was specified that a 100 per cent coverage is to be reached by 1983. To achieve this target, 3 million fly swotters were to be distributed every year.

(ix) Implementation of food and drugs act

The target was to correct the ignorance of the population concerning food hygiene and the handling of pesticides. CHP aimed at a total coverage of all local government areas in a period of 5 years.

(x) Use of pavements and enforcement of Highway Codes

A number of measures against road traffic accidents was taken: safe pedestrian crossings, better lighting of roads, use of seat belts and helmets, testing of vehicles *etc*. One aimed at covering the country by such measures within 5 years.

(xi) Detection and treatment of veneral diseases

The target was to cover all patients in 5 years. A number of suitable measures, such as blood testing of prostitutes and other high risk groups, was introduced.

The CHP for Sri Lanka contains a description of the problems in each critical area together with the possible solutions. For each area, *targets* were set, and *health development programs* were elaborated. CHP also stresses the need for integration in health planning of those institutions that are important in each of the priority areas. For instance, in the case of water supply, the National Water Supply and Drainage Board is responsible for the construction of water supply schemes. Local government institutions are responsible for the operation, maintenance and distribution of water supply schemes. It is imperative that the institutions mentioned collaborate within CHP to achieve the targets set.

To make CHP work better, the health administration framework was also adjusted. First, there is a National Health Development Council that is chaired by the Minister of Health. Secondly, District Health Councils and Division Health Councils were installed. The latter councils are to bring about a greater participation from the local population in health planning.

Three *constraints* are hampering the smooth implementation of CHP. First, there appears to be shortage of some categories of medical personnel such as public health nurses, food and drug inspectors, health educators, health officers, sanitary inspectors *etc*. Secondly, lack of transport inhibits the execution of CHP and makes supervision and communication with field workers rather difficult. Thirdly, the major problem seems to be a financial one. The health sector has to compete with other sectors for the country's scarce resources. Despite these problems, it is recognized that Sri Lanka is coming nearer to the various ambitious health targets it has set. In the coming years, it needs certainly to be investigated to what extent the CHP's targets have been completely achieved.

9.3. CHP AND ECONOMICS

9.3.1. CHP AND THE POPULATION'S PREFERENCES

In the second stage of CHP, health targets have to be set. According to us, it is important that targets are related as much as possible to people's preferences. In other words, we argue here in favor of a *bottom up* planning process, *i.e.* a process that starts from the health needs of the population and that counts on its participation. Such an approach differs from a *top down* planning process that is dominated by experts'opinions and preferences.

The sovereignty of the population in defining its preferences is also firmly embedded in economic theory. In the case of health care, the situation frequently occurs that health personnel is better informed (in a technical sense) about certain health problems and their causes than the population. One is therefore tempted to organize health interventions that are based on health personnel's knowledge and preferences. This is wrong in so far as the population would not understand or accept the health measures taken on its behalf. Consider the example of the use of clean water following upon the installation of a water pump. If people do not understand the importance of clean water for health, they are likely to make insufficient use or no use of it, making the decision about the water pump's installation very inadequate. In fact, the demand for clean water has to come mainly from the population itself. A better strategy would be to provide health education. The latter is not to be considered as an interference with people's preferences as such but rather as a transfer of information on health. This newly acquired knowledge is expected to entail a spontaneous demand for health measures. It is only in that case that health measures will have a lasting effect on people's health.

9.3.2. CHP AND ECONOMIC EVALUATION

In step 12 of the second stage of CHP, each health development program has to be confronted with a number of constraints. These constraints can be related to financing, manpower, equipment, logistics *etc.* The analysis of constraints is necessary so as to discard those programs that do not prove to be feasible.

In the third stage, one has to decide about the acceptance of the health development programs, that meet the constraints. Following upon the decision about those programs, one may have to decide, subsequently, about the health projects that evolve from the accepted programs. All these decisions can certainly be facilitated by the use of economic evaluation techniques.

It should be clear, however, that there is *no unique* evaluation method. The choice of the method will frequently be influenced by the health researchers' own preferences. If they are willing to measure health benefits and costs in monetary terms, they are likely to use CBA. If they want to achieve certain targets in a most efficient manner, they may turn to CEA. If they are interested in the multidimensional character of health, they will be attracted by MPA. If they intend to optimize a health objective, given a number of structural constraints, they may prefer to use LP. If they are concerned about the linkages between health and the economy, they may want to use RA. In a number of cases, the choice of evaluation method is dictated by the availability of information, however. Also note that the use of evaluation techniques *per se* is not to be aimed at. One should rather concentrate on the *results* of evaluation exercises in order to come nearer to predetermined health targets.

NOTES

[1] See WHO (1978). For earlier work on health planning, see Taylor (1972).
[2] See WHO (1978, p.10).
[3] This section relies heavily on WHO (1978).
[4] See WHO (1978, p.17).
[5] This subsection relies heavily on Orubuloye and Oyeneye (1982).

Appendix 1

PREVALENCE AND MORTALITY OF MAJOR DISEASES OF
AFRICA, ASIA AND LATIN AMERICA, 1977-1978

Infection	Infections thousands/year	Deaths thousands/year
Diarrhea	3-5,000,000	5-10,000
Malaria	800,000	1,200
Measles	85,000	900
Schistosomiasis	200,000	500 - 1,000
Tuberculosis	1,000,000	400
Hookworm	7,900,000	50 - 60
Onchocerciasis (river blindness)	30,000	20 - 50
Ascariasis (roundworm)	800,000-1,000,000	20
Typhoid	1,000	25
African Trypanoso-miasis (sleeping sickness)	1,000	5
Malnutrition	5 - 800,000	2,000

Source: Walsh and Warren (1979, p.968).

DATA ON GNP, HEALTH STATUS AND HEALTH DETERMINANTS

		Gross National Product per capita (dollars) (GNP) 1980	Life expectancy at birth (years) (LIFE)		Infant mortality rate (aged 0-1) (IM)		Child death rate (aged 1-4) (CD)		Crude death rate per thousand population (CRD)	
			1960	1980	1960	1980	1960	1980	1960	1980
Low-income economies										
1	Kampuchea,Dem.	..	46	..	146	..	22	..	19	..
2	Lao PDR	..	44	43	155	129	24	19	19	21
3	Bhutan	80	38	44	195	150	33	23	26	19
4	Chad	120	35	41	195	149	46	32	29	23
5	Bangladesh	130	37	46	159	136	25	20	28	18
6	Ethiopia	140	36	40	175	146	40	32	28	24
7	Nepal	140	38	44	195	150	33	23	27	20
8	Somalia	..	36	44	175	146	40	32	28	20
9	Burma	170	44	54	158	101	25	13	21	14
10	Afghanistan	..	33	37	233	205	41	35	31	26
11	Viet Nam	..	43	63	157	62	25	6	21	9
12	Mali	190	37	43	195	154	46	34	27	21
13	Burundi	200	37	42	150	122	33	25	27	22
14	Rwanda	200	37	45	147	137	32	29	27	20
15	Upper Volta	210	36	39	252	211	63	51	27	24
16	Zaire	220	40	47	150	112	33	22	24	18
17	Malawi	230	37	44	207	172	49	39	27	22
18	Mozambique	230	37	47	160	115	36	23	26	18
19	India	240	43	52	165	123	26	17	22	14
20	Haiti	270	44	53	182	115	47	18	20	14
21	Sri Lanka	270	62	66	71	44	7	3	9	7
22	Sierra Leone	280	37	47	234	208	57	50	27	18
23	Tanzania	280	42	52	152	103	33	19	22	15
24	China	290	..	64	..	56	..	5	14	8
25	Guinea	290	35	45	208	165	50	37	30	20
26	Central African Rep.	300	36	44	195	149	46	32	28	21
27	Pakistan	300	43	50	162	126	25	18	24	16
28	Uganda	300	44	54	139	97	29	18	20	14

Appendix 2 (cont'd')

	Gross National Product per capita (dollars) (GNP) 1980	Life expectancy at birth (years) (LIFE) 1960	1980	Infant mortality rate (aged 0-1) (IM) 1960	1980	Child death rate (aged 1-4) (CD) 1960	1980	Crude death rate per thousand population (CRD) 1960	1980
Low-income economies									
29 Benin	310	37	47	206	154	49	34	27	18
30 Niger	330	37	43	191	146	45	31	27	22
31 Madagascar	350	37	47	109	71	21	11	27	18
32 Sudan	410	40	46	168	124	40	22	25	19
33 Togo	410	37	47	182	109	42	21	27	18
Middle-income economies									
34 Ghana	420	40	49	143	103	31	19	24	17
35 Kenya	420	41	55	138	87	29	15	24	13
36 Lesotho	420	42	51	144	115	31	23	23	16
37 Yemen, PDR	420	36	45	209	146	59	31	29	20
38 Indonesia	430	41	53	150	93	23	11	23	13
39 Yeman Arab Rep.	430	36	42	212	190	60	50	29	23
40 Mauritania	440	37	43	185	143	43	31	27	22
41 Senegal	450	37	43	182	147	42	32	27	21
42 Angola	470	33	42	208	154	50	34	31	22
43 Liberia	530	44	54	194	154	46	34	21	14
44 Honduras	560	46	58	145	88	30	10	19	11
45 Zambia	560	40	49	151	106	33	20	24	17
46 Bolivia	570	43	50	167	131	40	25	22	16
47 Egypt	580	46	57	128	103	34	14	19	12
48 Zimbabwe	630	49	55	118	74	23	12	17	13
49 El Salvador	660	51	63	136	78	26	7	17	9
50 Cameroon	670	37	47	162	109	36	21	27	19
51 Thailand	670	52	63	103	55	13	4	15	8
52 Philippines	690	53	64	106	55	14	4	15	7
53 Nicaragua	740	47	56	144	91	30	10	19	12
54 Papua New Guin.	780	41	51	165	105	26	14	23	15
55 Congo, People's Rep.	900	48	59	171	129	39	27	18	10
56 Morocco	900	47	56	161	107	37	15	23	13
57 Mongolia	..	52	64	109	55	14	4	15	8
58 Albania	..	62	70	83	48	10	4	11	6
59 Peru	930	47	58	163	88	38	9	20	11
60 Nigeria	1010	39	49	183	135	42	28	25	17
61 Jamaica	1040	64	71	52	16	3	(.)	10	6
62 Guatemala	1080	47	59	92	70	10	6	19	11
63 Ivory Coast	1150	37	47	173	127	39	26	26	18
64 Dominican Rep.	1160	51	61	119	68	20	6	16	9
65 Colombia	1180	53	63	93	56	11	4	14	8
66 Ecuador	1270	51	61	140	82	28	8	17	10
67 Paraguay	1300	56	65	86	47	9	3	13	7
68 Tunisia	1310	48	60	159	90	36	10	21	9
69 Korea,Dem.Rep.	..	54	65	78	34	9	2	13	7
70 Syrian Arab.Rep.	1340	50	65	132	62	25	5	18	8
71 Jordan	1420	47	61	136	69	26	6	20	10
72 Lebanon	..	58	66	68	41	5	2	14	8
73 Turkey	1470	51	62	190	123	50	21	16	10

Appendix 2 (cont'd')

	Gross National Product per capita (dollars) (GNP)	Life expectancy at birth (years) (LIFE)		Infant mortality rate (aged 0-1) (IM)		Child death rate (aged 1-4) (CD)		Crude death rate per thousand population (CRD)	
	1980	1960	1980	1960	1980	1960	1980	1960	1980
74 Cuba	..	63	73	66	21	5	1	9	6
75 Korea,Rep.of	1520	54	65	78	34	9	2	13	7
76 Malaysia	1620	53	64	72	31	7	2	16	7
77 Costa Rica	1730	62	70	71	24	6	1	10	5
78 Panama	1730	62	70	68	22	5	1	10	6
79 Algeria	1870	47	56	165	118	39	19	23	13
80 Brazil	2050	55	63	118	77	19	7	13	9
81 Mexico	2090	58	65	91	56	10	4	12	7
82 Chile	2150	57	67	114	43	18	2	12	7
83 South Africa	2300	53	61	135	96	28	18	15	10
84 Romania	2340	65	71	69	29	7	2	9	10
85 Portugal	2370	63	71	81	35	9	2	8	10
86 Argentina	2390	65	70	61	45	4	2	9	8
87 Yugoslavia	2620	63	70	92	33	11	2	10	9
88 Uruguay	2810	68	71	50	40	3	2	9	10
89 Iran	..	50	59	163	108	26	14	17	11
90 Iraq	3020	46	56	139	78	28	7	20	12
91 Venezuela	3630	57	67	85	42	9	2	11	6
92 Hong Kong	4240	67	74	42	13	3	(.)	8	5
93 Trinidad and Tobago	4370	64	72	45	24	2	1	9	5
94 Greece	4380	69	74	40	19	3	1	8	10
95 Singapore	4430	64	72	36	12	2	1	8	5
96 Israel	4500	69	72	32	14	1	(.)	6	7
High-income oil exporters									
97 Libya	8640	47	56	158	100	36	13	19	12
98 Saudi Arabia	11260	43	54	185	114	48	18	23	14
99 Kuwait	19830	60	70	89	34	10	1	10	5
100 Un.Arab Emirates	26850	47	63	135	53	26	3	19	7

Appendix 2 (cont'd')

	Percentage of population with access to safe water (ASW) 1975	Population per physician (PHY)		Population per nursing person (NUR)		Adult literacy rate (per cent) (LIT)		Daily per capita calorie supply as percentage of requirement (CAL)		Total fertility rate (FERT)		Crude birth rate per thousand population (CRB)	
	1975	1960	1977	1960	1977	1960	1977	1974	1977	1975	1980	1960	1980
Low-income economies													
1 Kampuchea, Dem.	..	35,440	..	4,010	..	36	..	85	78	6.7	..	45	..
2 Lao PDR	..	53,520	20,060	4,950	3,040	28	41	93	94	6.2	6.1	42	42
3 Bhutan	..	..	..	5,780	..	..	..	94	90	6.2	5.5	43	39
4 Chad	26	72,190	41,940	..	3,820	6	15	75	72	5.3	5.9	45	44
5 Bangladesh	53	..	12,690	..	40,490	22	26	92	..	6.6	6.0	54	45
6 Ethiopia	6	100,470	74,910	14,920	5,320	..	15	82	78	6.7	6.7	51	49
7 Nepal	9	73,800	35,900	..	13,510	9	19	95	89	6.2	6.1	44	42
8 Somalia	33	36,570	18,480	8,810	..	2	60	79	88	6.1	6.1	47	46
9 Burma	17	15,560	5,260	8,550	4,400	60	70	103	103	5.5	5.3	43	37
10 Afghanistan	6	28,700	20,550	19,590	25,920	8	12	83	107	6.9	6.6	50	47
11 Viet Nam	..	..	5,620	..	2,470	..	87	111	96	6.2	5.2	47	36
12 Mali	9	67,050	25,560	4,920	2,380	3	9	75	83	6.7	6.7	50	50
13 Burundi	..	96,570	45,020	4,530	6,180	14	23	99	99	6.3	6.4	47	46
14 Rwanda	35	143,290	38,790	11,620	10,460	16	50	90	94	6.9	8.3	51	53
15 Upper Volta	25	81,650	50,000	4,090	3,650	2	5	78	93	6.5	6.5	49	48
16 Zaire	16	37,620	15,530	3,510	1,620	31	58	85	102	5.9	6.1	48	46
17 Malawi	33	35,250	41,010	12,920	3,830	..	25	103	97	6.1	7.8	53	56
18 Mozambique	..	20,390	35,820	4,720	4,290	11	28	84	78	5.7	6.1	46	45
19 India	33	4,850	3,630	10,980	5,700	28	36	89	89	5.7	4.9	44	36
20 Haiti	14	9,230	5,940	4,020	2,940	15	23	90	92	4.9	4.8	39	36
21 Sri Lanka	20	4,490	6,700	4,170	2,040	75	85	91	97	4.2	3.6	36	28
22 Sierra Leone	..	20,420	..	2,960	..	7	..	97	85	5.9	6.1	47	46
23 Tanzania	39	18,220	17,550	11,890	2,390	10	66	86	87	6.7	6.5	47	46

Appendix 2 (cont'd')

	Percentage of population with access to safe water (ASW) 1975	Population per physician (PHY) 1960	(PHY) 1977	Population per nursing person (NUR) 1960	(NUR) 1977	Adult literacy rate (per cent) (LIT) 1960	(LIT) 1977	Daily per capita calorie supply as percentage of requirement (CAL) 1974	(CAL) 1977	Total fertility rate (FERT) 1975	(FERT) 1980	Crude birth rate per thousand population (CRB) 1960	(CRB) 1980
24 China	..	3,010	1,100	2,850	480	.7	66	99	103	3.8	2.9	40	21
25 Guinea	10	26,900	16,630	3,260	2,490	7	20	84	78	6.2	6.2	47	46
26 Central African Rep.	16	49,610	20,280	3,280	1,540	7	39	102	92	5.5	5.9	43	44
27 Pakistan	29	5,400	3,780	16,960	10,030	15	24	93	99	7.2	6.1	51	44
28 Uganda	35	15,050	26,810	10,030	4,180	35	48	90	93	6.1	6.1	45	45
29 Benin	21	23,030	26,570	2,690	2,360	5	25	87	100	6.7	7.1	51	49
30 Niger	27	82,170	42,720	8,460	2,380	1	5	78	91	7.1	7.1	52	52
31 Madagascar	25	8,900	10,240	3,110	2,300	..	50	105	111	6.7	6.5	47	47
32 Sudan	46	33,420	8,780	3,030	850	13	20	88	96	7.0	6.7	47	47
33 Togo	16	35,760	18,160	5,340	1,740	10	18	96	92	6.7	6.5	51	48
Middle-income economies													
34 Ghana	35	21,600	9,920	5,430	610	27	..	101	85	6.7	6.7	49	48
35 Kenya	17	10,690	11,630	2,270	1,090	20	50	91	96	7.6	7.8	52	51
36 Lesotho	17	23,490	18,640	..	14,900	..	52	99	95	5.1	5.8	41	43
37 Yemen, PDR	24	13,290	5,970	..	1,330	..	40	84	81	7.2	6.7	50	46
38 Indonesia	12	46,780	13,670	4,520	8,870	39	62	98	102	5.5	4.5	46	35
39 Yemen Arab.Rep.	4	130,010	11,670	..	4,580	3	21	83	82	7.2	6.5	50	47
40 Mauritania	..	37,040	13,700	4,980	1,980	5	17	72	94	5.9	6.9	51	50
41 Senegal	37	21,970	15,710	2,840	1,390	6	10	97	95	6.3	6.5	48	48
42 Angola	..	14,910	..	6,570	..	.9	..	86	93	6.5	6.4	50	48
43 Liberia	20	12,600	9,280	1,410	1,810	.9	25	87	101	5.7	6.9	50	49
44 Honduras	46	12,610	3,290	..	870	45	60	90	93	7.3	6.8	51	45
45 Zambia	42	9,540	10,410	9,920	1,970	29	44	90	90	6.9	6.9	51	49
46 Bolivia	34	3,830	1,850	..	3,070	39	63	77	87	6.2	6.1	46	43
47 Egypt	66	2,560	1,050	1,930	1,100	26	44	113	118	5.2	4.9	44	37

48 Zimbabwe	..	4,790	7,030	1,010	1,170	39	74	108	109	6.6	8.0	55	54
49 El Salvador	53	5,260	3,600	..	950	49	62	84	94	6.2	5.7	49	41
50 Cameroon	26	48,110	16,500	3,280	1,150	19	..	102	106	5.5	5.5	43	42
51 Thailand	22	7,950	8,220	4,860	1,170	68	84	107	97	6.3	4.0	44	30
52 Philippines	43	..	2,810	..	3,170	72	75	87	107	6.4	4.6	46	34
53 Nicaragua	70	2,690	1,590	1,250	800	..	90	105	116	6.9	6.3	51	45
54 Papua New Guinea	20	14,390	14,040	2,450	1,590	29	32	98	87	6.0	5.2	44	37
55 Congo People's Rep.	17	16,100	7,470	1,300	600	16	..	98	99	5.8	6.0	40	42
56 Morocco	..	9,410	11,040	..	1,830	14	28	108	107	7.1	6.5	52	44
57 Mongolia	..	1,070	480	300	250	..	..	102	106	5.6	5.2	41	35
58 Albania	..	3,630	960	530	320	..	80	105	113	4.9	3.9	41	30
59 Peru	48	2,010	1,530	2,210	680	61	80	100	98	5.8	5.0	47	36
60 Nigeria	..	73,710	15,740	4,040	2,880	15	30	88	83	6.7	6.9	52	50
61 Jamaica	86	2,590	3,520	1,990	550	82	90	119	118	5.4	3.9	39	29
62 Guatemala	40	4,420	2,560	9,040	..	32	..	91	92	6.1	5.4	48	40
63 Ivory Coast	19	29,190	21,040	2,920	1,590	5	41	115	107	6.2	6.7	50	47
64 Dominican Republic	55	8,220	1,970	..	..	65	67	98	102	6.9	4.8	50	36
65 Colombia	64	2,640	1,570	4,220	1,250	63	..	94	98	5.9	3.8	46	30
66 Ecuador	42	2,670	2,190	2,360	..	68	81	93	90	6.3	6.0	47	40
67 Paraguay	13	1,810	..	..	2,290	75	84	118	119	6.2	4.9	43	36
68 Tunisia	70	10,030	3,580	..	1,070	16	62	102	115	6.2	5.4	49	35
69 Korea, Dem.Rep.	..	..	..	6,660	..	..	..	113	119	5.2	4.3	42	31
70 Syrian Arab.Rep.	75	4,630	2,570	1,930	3,900	30	58	104	104	7.1	7.0	47	45
71 Jordan	61	5,800	1,960	2,080	820	32	70	90	62	7.1	6.9	47	44
72 Lebanon	..	1,210	..	..	..	..	..	101	112	6.3	4.1	43	30
73 Turkey	75	3,000	1,760	..	920	38	60	113	116	5.8	4.4	43	32
74 Cuba	..	1,060	1,100	950	..	..	96	117	118	4.0	2.2	32	18
75 Korea Rep.of	71	3,540	1,980	3,250	490	71	93	112	117	4.0	3.0	43	24
76 Malaysia	62	7,020	7,640	1,790	870	53	..	115	116	5.7	4.2	45	31
77 Costa Rica	77	2,700	1,390	710	450	..	90	113	113	4.6	3.4	47	29
78 Panama	79	2,730	1,220	3,460	1,410	73	..	105	104	5.1	3.9	41	31
79 Algeria	77	5,530	5,330	..	1,480	10	35	88	97	7.2	6.9	50	46

Appendix 2 (cont'd)

	Percentage of population with access to safe water (ASW) 1975	Population per physician (PHY) 1960	(PHY) 1977	Population per nursing person (NUR) 1960	(NUR) 1977	Adult literacy rate (per cent) (LIT) 1960	(LIT) 1977	Daily per capita calorie supply as percentage of requirement (CAL) 1974	(CAL) 1977	Total fertility rate (FERT) 1975	(FERT) 1980	Crude birth rate per thousand population (CRB) 1960	(CRB) 1980
80 Brazil	77	2,560	1,700	2,770	822	61	76	105	111	5.2	4.1	43	30
81 Mexico	62	1,820	1,260	3,630	1,420	65	81	117	113	6.5	5.1	45	37
82 Chile	84	1,780	1,930	640	420	84	..	117	110	3.7	2.8	37	22
83 South Africa	..	2,180	..	480	..	57	..	118	116	5.6	5.1	39	38
84 Romania	..	790	740	620	470	89	98	123	130	2.6	2.5	20	18
85 Portugal	65	1,250	700	1,420	470	62	..	141	127	2.6	2.4	24	18
86 Argentina	66	740	530	750	..	91	93	129	124	3.0	2.8	24	21
87 Yugoslavia	..	1,620	760	630	360	77	85	136	136	2.4	2.2	24	17
88 Uruguay	84	970	540	..	3,700	..	94	116	105	2.9	2.8	22	20
89 Iran	51	4,060	2,560	8,090	1,900	16	50	98	122	6.9	5.8	46	41
90 Iraq	62	5,270	2,190	3,030	1,890	18	..	101	90	7.1	6.6	49	45
91 Venezuela	..	1,510	930	2,840	370	63	82	98	102	5.3	4.5	46	35
92 Hong Kong	..	3,060	1,180	2,880	430	70	90	110	119	3.0	2.2	35	17
93 Trinidad and Tobago	..	2,390	1,970	750	580	93	95	105	103	3.4	2.6	38	23
94 Greece	..	800	460	800	600	81	..	132	135	2.3	2.3	19	16
95 Singapore	100	2,360	1,250	650	380	..	..	122	135	2.8	1.8	38	17
96 Israel	..	400	310	360	..	84	..	122	123	3.7	3.4	27	24
High-income oil-exporters													
97 Libya	100	6,580	900	1,320	350	22	..	117	122	6.8	7.0	49	45
98 Saudi Arabia	84	16,370	1,700	5,850	860	3	16	102	87	7.2	6.9	49	44
99 Kuwait	89	1,150	790	260	230	47	60	..	..	7.2	6.1	44	39
100 Un.Arab Emirates	..	..	..	..	430	..	56	..	..	..	6.4	46	28

Source: Statistical Appendix, World Bank (1982). Exceptions are CAL (1974) and LIT (1975); they are taken from the Statistical Appendix of World Bank (1979) and World Bank (1978) respectively. It must be mentioned that some figures are for other years than those specified; see the original sources for more details.

Notes: .. means not available.
(.) means less than half the unit shown.

Appendix 3

ELEMENTS OF DESCRIPTIVE STATISTICS

3.1. FREQUENCY DISTRIBUTION

Suppose one has a certain amount of information, say n observations, about a variable x. One can now define a number of *intervals* and compute the number of times values of x are located in those intervals. This will result in a *frequency distribution* of x. The frequencies obtained can be divided by n in order to compute the *relative frequencies* of the data. The frequency distribution can also be depicted graphically by a *histogram*, in which one can use bars to represent relative frequencies.

3.2. MEASURES OF LOCATION AND SPREAD

(i) The most popular measure of *location* or of *central tendency* is the *mean*. One sums the n observation of x and divides by n; namely

$$\bar{x} = \frac{\sum\limits_{i=1}^{n} x_i}{n}$$

where x_i refers to the i-th observation of x. The mean $\bar{x}$ may be viewed as the center or balancing point of the data.

(ii) The simplest measure of *spread* is the *range*. It is equal to the maximum value minus the minimum value of the data. However, the range gives no information about the dispersion of the observations between these extremes. A measure that takes account of all data is the *variance*[1]; it is equal to

$$\sigma_x^2 = \frac{1}{n-1} \sum_i^n (x_i - \bar{x})^2$$

One obtains another measure of spread by taking the square root of the variance. This measure is called the *standard deviation* of x:

$$\sigma_x = \sqrt{\frac{1}{n-1} \sum_i^n (x_i - \bar{x})^2}$$

Note that the standard deviation has the same dimension as the variable x.

Whereas the standard deviation measures absolute dispersion around the mean, a measure of *relative dispersion* is the *coefficient of variation:*

$$C = \frac{\sigma_x}{\bar{x}}$$

An advantage of the coefficient of variation is that it is independent of the unit used.

(iii) Certainly not all frequency distributions are symmetric around a single peak. It may happen that they have a longer tail to the right of the mean than to the left. One then says that these distributions are *skewed to the right* or that they have *positive skewness*. Distributions with *negative skewness* have a longer tail to the left of the mean; they are *skewed to the left*. A measure of skewness frequently used is the following

$$skewness = \frac{\frac{1}{n} \sum_i^n (x_i - \bar{x})^3}{\sigma_x^3}$$

For perfectly symmetrical distributions, this skewness coefficient is zero. It is positive and negative in the case of positive and negative skewness respectively.

(iv) When studying frequency distributions, one may wish to know the degree of their *peakedness*. Usually this peakedness is measured relative to the *normal distribution*[2]. The measure of this relative degree of peakedness is called the kurtosis and is computed as follows:

$$kurtosis = \frac{\frac{1}{n} \sum_{i}^{n} (x_i - \bar{x})^4}{\sigma_x^4} - 3$$

For normal distributions, the kurtosis can be proven to be zero. For a distribution[3] that is broader than the bell shaped normal curve, the kurtosis is less than 0. Such a distribution is called *platy-kurtic*. The kurtosis will exceed 0 for a distribution that is narrower than the normal curve. In that case the curve is called *leptokurtic*.

In Figure A3.1, examples are given of differently skewed and peaked continuous probability density curves.

NOTES

[1] One divides by n-1 in order to obtain an un-biased estimate of the population variance; see Wonnacott and Wonnacott (1969, ch.2).
[2] The normal distribution is widely used in statistics. It is a continuous curve that is bell shaped; see Figure A3.1.
[3] Note that for a very large amount of data only, a frequency distribution can be converted in-to a continuous probability density curve. See Wonnacott and Wonnacott (1969, pp.63-71).

Figure A3.1. Different shapes of continuous
probability density curves

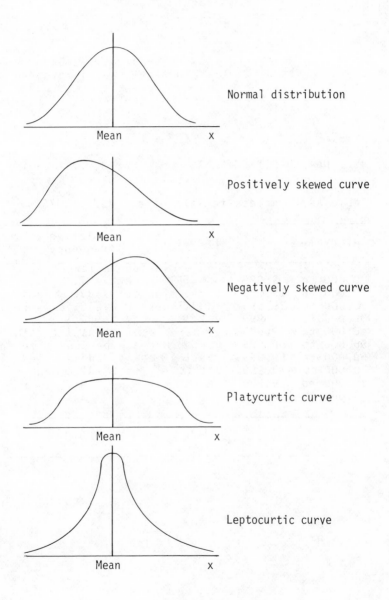

Normal distribution

Positively skewed curve

Negatively skewed curve

Platycurtic curve

Leptocurtic curve

Appendix 4

FREQUENCY DISTRIBUTIONS

4.1. HEALTH DETERMINANTS

Table A4.1. Access to safe water (ASW), 1975

Interval	Frequency	Relative frequency
0.000 to 9.999	5	7.1
10.000 to 19.999	12	17.1
20.000 to 29.999	12	17.1
30.000 to 39.999	9	12.9
40.000 to 49.999	7	10.0
50.000 to 59.999	4	5.7
60.000 to 69.999	8	11.4
70.000 to 79.999	9	12.9
80.000 to 89.999	3	4.3
90.000 to 100.000	1	1.4
TOTAL	70	100.0

Table A4.2. Population per physician (PHY)

Interval			Frequency		Relative frequency	
			1960	1977	1960	1977
0.000	to	1999.999	13	29	15.3	34.1
2000.000	to	2999.999	11	5	12.9	5.9
3000.000	to	3999.999	6	6	7.1	7.1
4000.000	to	4999.999	6	0	7.1	0.0
5000.000	to	9999.999	11	12	12.9	14.1
10000.000	to	14999.999	6	8	7.1	9.4
15000.000	to	19999.999	4	9	4.7	10.6
20000.000	to	29999.999	8	7	9.4	8.2
30000.000	to	39999.999	6	3	7.1	3.5
40000.000	to	144000.000	14	6	16.5	7.1
TOTAL			85	85	100.0	100.0

Table A4.3. Population per nurse (NUR)

Interval			Frequency		Relative frequency	
			1960	1977	1960	1977
0.000	to	1999.999	19	42	28.8	63.6
2000.000	to	3999.999	20	14	30.3	21.2
4000.000	to	5999.999	15	5	22.7	7.6
6000.000	to	7999.999	1	1	1.5	1.5
8000.000	to	9999.999	4	1	6.1	1.5
10000.000	to	11999.999	3	2	4.5	3.0
12000.000	to	13999.999	1	0	1.5	0.0
14000.000	to	15999.999	1	0	1.5	0.0
16000.000	to	17999.999	1	0	1.5	0.0
18000.000	to	26000.000	1	1	1.5	1.5
TOTAL			66	66	100.0	100.0

Frequency distributions

Table A4.4. Adult literacy (%) (LIT)

Interval	Frequency		Relative frequency	
	1960	1977	1960	1977
0.000 to 9.999	15	3	23.8	4.8
10.000 to 19.999	13	6	20.6	9.5
20.000 to 29.999	7	11	11.1	17.5
30.000 to 39.999	8	5	12.7	7.9
40.000 to 49.999	2	5	3.2	7.9
50.000 to 59.999	0	5	0.0	7.9
60.000 to 69.999	8	9	12.7	14.3
70.000 to 79.999	6	5	9.5	7.9
80.000 to 89.999	2	8	3.2	12.7
90.000 to 100.000	2	6	3.2	9.5
TOTAL	63	63	100.0	100.0

Table A4.5. Daily per capita calorie supply as percentage of requirement (CAL)

Interval	Frequency		Relative frequency	
	1974	1977	1974	1977
60.000 to 69.999	0	1	0.0	1.1
70.000 to 79.999	7	5	7.4	5.3
80.000 to 89.999	18	12	18.9	12.6
90.000 to 99.999	27	31	28.4	32.6
100.000 to 109.999	20	19	21.1	20.0
110.000 to 119.999	16	19	16.8	20.0
120.000 to 129.999	4	4	4.2	4.2
130.000 to 139.999	2	4	2.1	4.2
140.000 to 145.000	1	0	1.1	0.0
TOTAL	95	95	100.0	100.0

Table A4.6. Fertility rate (FERT)

Interval	Frequency		Relative frequency	
	1975	1980	1975	1980
1.000 to 1.999	0	1	0.0	1.1
2.000 to 2.999	6	11	6.3	11.6
3.000 to 3.999	6	8	6.3	8.4
4.000 to 4.999	6	14	6.3	14.7
5.000 to 5.999	25	16	26.3	16.8
6.000 to 6.999	40	39	42.1	41.1
7.000 to 7.999	12	4	12.6	4.2
8.000 to 9.000	0	2	0.0	2.1
TOTAL	95	95	100.0	100.0

Table A4.7. Crude birth rate per thousand population
          (CRB)

Interval	Frequency		Relative frequency	
	1960	1980	1960	1980
15.000 to 19.999	1	7	1.1	7.4
20.000 to 24.999	5	7	5.3	7.4
25.000 to 29.999	1	3	1.1	3.2
30.000 to 34.999	1	10	1.1	10.5
35.000 to 39.999	8	16	8.4	16.8
40.000 to 44.999	22	15	23.2	15.8
45.000 to 49.999	32	29	33.7	30.5
50.000 to 54.999	24	7	25.3	7.4
55.000 to 60.000	1	1	1.1	1.1
TOTAL	95	95	100.0	100.0

4.2. HEALTH STATUS

Table A4.8. Crude death rate per thousand
population (CRD)

Interval	Frequency		Relative frequency	
	1960	1980	1960	1980
5.000 to 9.999	11	31	11.6	32.6
10.000 to 14.999	15	26	15.8	27.4
15.000 to 19.999	18	19	18.9	20.0
20.000 to 24.999	22	18	23.2	18.9
25.000 to 29.999	26	1	27.4	1.1
30.000 to 35.000	3	0	3.2	0.0
TOTAL	95	95	100.0	100.0

Table A4.9. Life expectancy at birth in years
(LIFE)

Interval	Frequency		Relative frequency	
	1960	1980	1960	1980
30.000 to 34.999	2	0	2.1	0.0
35.000 to 39.999	26	2	27.7	2.1
40.000 to 44.999	18	15	19.1	16.0
45.000 to 44.999	12	16	12.8	17.0
50.000 to 54.999	14	11	14.9	11.7
55.000 to 59.999	6	12	6.4	12.8
60.000 to 64.999	10	14	10.6	14.9
65.000 to 69.999	6	9	6.4	9.6
70.000 to 75.000	0	15	0.0	16.0
TOTAL	94	94	100.0	100.0

Table A4.10. Infant mortality, age 0-1 (IM)

Interval	Frequency		Relative frequency	
	1960	1980	1960	1980
10.000 to 49.999	5	23	5.3	24.5
50.000 to 89.999	16	19	17.0	20.2
90.000 to 129.999	13	28	13.8	29.8
130.000 to 169.999	34	19	36.2	20.2
170.000 to 209.999	22	4	23.4	4.3
210.000 to 249.999	3	1	3.2	1.1
250.000 to 255.000	1	0	1.1	0.0
TOTAL	94	94	100.0	100.0

Table A4.11. Child death rate, age 1-4 (CD)

Interval	Frequency		Relative frequency	
	1960	1980	1960	1980
0.000 to 4.999	5	25	5.5	27.5
5.000 to 9.999	12	10	13.2	11.0
10.000 to 14.999	8	10	8.8	11.0
15.000 to 19.999	2	11	2.2	12.1
20.000 to 24.999	5	11	5.5	12.1
25.000 to 29.999	15	6	16.5	6.6
30.000 to 34.999	12	12	13.2	13.2
35.000 to 39.999	8	3	8.8	3.3
40.000 to 44.999	9	0	9.9	0.0
45.000 to 65.000	15	3	16.5	3.3
TOTAL	91	91	100.0	100.0

Appendix 5

BASIC NEEDS MODEL: LIST OF COUNTRIES

1. Chad	27.*Indonesia
2. Ethiopia	28. Yemen A.R.
3.*Nepal	29. Senegal
4. Burma	30. Liberia
5.*Afghanistan	31.*Honduras
6. Mali	32. Zambia
7. Rwanda	33. Bolivia
8. Upper Volta	34.*Egypt
9. Zaire	35.*El Salvador
10. Malawi	36.*Thailand
11.*India	37.*Philippines
12.*Haiti	38.*Nicaragua
13.*Sri Lanka	39.*Papua N.G.
14. Tanzania	40. Peru
15. Guinea	41. Ivory Coast
16. Central African Republic	42.*Paragua
17.*Pakistan	43.*Tunisia
18. Uganda	44. Syrian A.R.
19. Benin	45.*Turkey
20. Niger	46.*Korea Rep. of
21. Madagascar	47.*Costa Rica
22. Sudan	48. Algeria
23. Togo	49. Brazil
24. Kenya	50.*Mexico
25. Lesotho	51. Uruguay
26. Yemen P.D.R.	

Note: The starred numbers refer to the countries
whose data are used in the estimation of the
equation for CRB and CONTRA.

FURTHER SELECTED READINGS

Chapters 1 and 2:

Lee, K. and A. Mills, *The Economics of Health in Developing Countries* (Oxford University Press, Oxford, 1983)
Sorkin, A.L. *Health Economics in Developing Countries* (Lexington Books, Lexington Mass., 1976)

Chapters 3 and 4:

Dasgupta, A.K. and D.W. Pierce, *Cost-Benefit Analysis - Theory and Practice* (MacMillan Press, London, 1978)
Drummond, M.F. *Principles of Economic Appraisal in Health Care* (Oxford University Press, Oxford, 1981)
—— *Studies in Economic Appraisal in Health Care* (Oxford University Press, Oxford, 1981)
Holland, W.H. (ed.) *Evaluation of Health Care* (Oxford University Press, Oxford, 1983)
Mooney, G.H., E.M. Russell and R.D. Weir, *Choices for Health Care* (The MacMillan Press, London, 1980)
Unido, *Guidelines for Project Evaluation* (United Nations, New York, 1972)

Chapter 5:

Keeney, R. and H. Raiffa, *Decisions with Multiple Objectives: Preferences and Value Tradeoffs*, (John Wiley, New York, 1976)

Further selected readings

Chapter 6:

Budnick, F.S., R. Mojena and T.E. Vollman, *Principles of Operations Research for Management* (Irwin Inc., Homewood Ill., 1977), chapters 4 to 10

Chiang, A. *Fundamental Methods of Mathematical Economics* (McGraw Hill, New York, 1967), chapters 18 and 19

Chapters 7 and 8:

Intriligator, M. *Econometric Models, Techniques and Applications* (North Holland, Amsterdam, 1978)

Kilpatrick, S.J. *Statistical Principles in Health Care Information* (University Park Press, Baltimore, MD, 1977)

Wonnacott, R.J. and T.H. Wonnacott, *Econometrics* (Wiley, New York, 1970)

Chapter 9:

Caldwell, H.R. and D.W. Dunlop, 'An Empirical Study of Health Planning in Latin America and Africa', *Social Science and Medecine*, vol. 13 C, (1979), pp.75-86

Reinke, W.A. (ed.) *Health Planning - Qualitative Aspects and Quantitative Techniques* (Waverley Press Inc., Baltimore, MD, 1972)

BIBLIOGRAPHY

Acton, J.P. 'Measuring the Social Impact of Heart and Circulatory Disease Programs: Preliminary Framework and Estimates', (Report R-1697-NHLI, Rand Corp., S.Monica, 1975)

Anker, R. and J.C. Knowles, *An Empirical Analysis of Mortality Differentials in Kenya at the Macro Level* (mimeo, 1977)

Azurin, J.C. and M. Alvero, 'Field Evaluation of Environmental Sanitation Measures Against Cholera', *Bulletin of the WHO*, vol.51, no.1 (1974), pp.19-26

Bainbridge, J. and S. Sapirie, *Health Project Management: A Manual of Procedures for Formulating and Implementing Health Projects* (WHO,Geneva, 1974)

Barlow, R. 'The Economic Effects of Malaria Eradication', *American Economic Review*, vol.LVII,no.2 (1967), pp.130-148

Barlow, R. 'Health and Economic Development: A Theoretical and Empirical Review' in I. Sirageldin (ed.), *Research in Human Capital and Development* (JAI Press, Greenwich, Connecticut, 1979)

Barnum, H. 'The Economic Costs and Benefits of an Immunization Program in Indonesia' (Discussion Paper no.89, Center for Research on Economic Development, Ann Arbor, 1981)

Barten, A.P. 'Methodological Aspects of Macroeconomic Model Construction' (Lecture notes, Cabay, Leuven, 1981)

Basta, S.S. and A. Churchill, 'Iron Deficiency Anaemia and the Productivity of Adult Males in Indonesia' (World Bank Staff Working Paper no. 175, World Bank, Washington D.C., 1974)

Baumol, W.J. *Economic Theory and Operations Analysis*, 4th edn (Prentice Hall, Englewood Cliffs,N.J., 1977)

Behrman, J.P. and B.L. Wolfe, *The Impact of Health and Nutrition on the Number of Surviving Children in a Developing Metropolis* (mimeo, 1979)

Berelson, B., W.P. Mauldin and S.J. Segal, 'Population: Current Status and Policy Options', *Social Science & Medecine*, vol. 14 C, (1980), pp.77-97

Berg, A., N.S. Scrimshaw and D.L. Call, *Nutrition, National Development and Planning* (M.I.T.Press, Cambridge, 1973)

Briscoe, J. 'The Role of Water Supply in Improving Health in Poor Countries' (with special reference to Bangladesh), *The American Journal of Clinical Nutrition*, vol.31, (1978), pp.2100-2113

Broome, J. 'Trying to Value a Life', *Journal of Public Economics*, vol.9, no.1 (1978), pp.91-100

Budnick, F.S., R. Mojena and T.E. Vollman, *Principles of Operations Research for Management* (Irwin Inc, Homewood Ill., 1977)

Chandra, R.K. 'Prospective Studies of the Effect of Breast-Feeding on Incidence of Infection and Allergy', *Acta Paediatrica Scandinavica*, no. 68 (1979)

Chernichovsky, D.'The Economic Theory of the Household and Impact Measurement of Nutrition and Related Health Programs' in R.E. Klein (ed.), *Evaluating the Impact of Nutrition and Health Programs* (Plenum Publishing Corporation, New York, 1979), pp.227-267

Chiang, A. *Fundamental Methods of Mathematical Economics* (McGraw Hill, New York, 1967)

Chowdhury, A.K.M.A. 'A Study of Neonatal and Post-Neonatal Differentials in Rural Bangladesh' (Master's thesis, Baltimore, The Johns Hopkins University, 1974)

Christiansen, N., *et.al.* 'Social Environment as It Relates to Malnutrition and Mental Development' in J. Cravioto, *et.al.* (eds.), *Early Malnutrition and Mental Development* (The Swedish Nutrition Foundation, Stockholm, 1974)

Clugston, G.A. 'The Effect of Malnutrition on Brain Growth and Intellectual Development' *Tropical Doctor*, vol.11, no.1 (1981), pp.32-38

Cochrane, S.H.,*et.al.* 'The Effects of Education on Health' (World Bank Staff Working Paper no.405, World Bank, Washington D.C., 1980)

Conly, G.N. 'The Impact of Malaria on Economic Development: a Case Study' (PAHO Scientific Publication no.297, PAHO, Washington D.C., 1975)

Cravioto, J. and E.L. Delicardie, 'Longitudinal Study of Language Development in Severely Malnourished Children' in G. Serban (ed.), *Nutrition and Mental Functions*(Plenum Press, New York, 1975)

Cullis, J.G. and P.A. West, *The Economics of Health* (Martin Robertson, London, 1979)

Curlin, G.T.,*et.al.* 'The Influence of Drinking Tubewell Water on Diarrhea Rates in Matlab Thana, Bangladesh' (Working Paper no.1, Cholera Research Laboratory, Dacca, 1977)

Dasgupta, A.K. and D.W. Pierce,*Cost-Benefit Analysis - Theory and Practice* (MacMillan Press, London, 1978)

Djukanovic, V. and E.P. Mach (eds.), *Alternative Approaches to Meeting Basic Health Needs in Developing Countries* (WHO and UNICEF, Geneva,1975)

Dunlop D.W. 'A Linear Programming Approach to Health Planning in Developing Countries with an Application in East Africa' (Discussion paper, Darthmouth Medical School, August 1982)

Feldstein M.S. 'The Inadequacy of Weighted Discount Rates' in R. Layard (ed.), *Cost-Benefit Analysis* (Penguin Books Inc, Harmondsworth, Middlesex, 1972)

Gopalan, C. and V.K. Rao, 'Nutrition and Family Size', *Journal of Nutrition and Diet*, vol.6, no.3 (1969), pp.258-266

Graves, P.L. 'Nutrition and Infant Behavior: A Replication Study in the Kathmandu Valley, Nepal', *American Journal of Clinical Nutrition*, vol.31, (1978), pp.541-551

Gray, R.H. 'The Decline of Malaria Mortality in Ceylon and the Demographic Effects of Malaria Control', *Population Studies*, vol.28, (1974), pp. 205-229

Grosse, R.N. 'Interrelation between Health and Population: Observations Derived from Field Experiences', *Social Science & Medecine*, vol.14 C, no.2 (1980), pp.99-120

Grosse, R.N., J.L. de Vries, R.L. Tilden, A. Dievler and R.S. Day, 'A Health Development Model - Application to Rural Java' (Final Report prepared for the Bureau for Program and Policy Co-ordination, U.S. Agency for International Development, The University of Michigan, Ann Arbor, 1979)

Gwatkin, D.R.,*et.al.* 'Can Health and Nutrition Interventions Make a Difference?' (Monograph no.13, Overseas Development Council, Washington D.C., 1980)

Heller, P. 'Issues in the Costing of Public Sector Outputs: The Public Medical Services of Malay-

sia' (World Bank Staff Paper no.207, World
    Bank, Washington D.C., 1975)
Hicks, N. 'Economic Growth and Human Resources'
    (World Bank Staff Paper no.408, World Bank,
    Washington D.C., 1980)
Hirshleifer, J. *Price Theory and Applications*
    (Prentice Hall, Englewood Cliffs N.J., 1976)
Hu, T.W. 'The Financing and the Economic Efficiency
    of Rural Health Services in the People's Repub-
    lic of China', *International Journal of Health
    Services*, vol.6, no.2 (1976), pp.239-249
Intriligator, M. *Mathematical Optimization and Eco-
    nomic Theory* (Prentice Hall, Englewood Cliffs,
    N.J., 1971)
—— *Econometric Models, Techniques and Applications*
    (North Holland, Amsterdam, 1978)
Isenman, P. 'Basic Needs: the Case of Sri Lanka',
    World Development, vol.8, (1980), pp.237-258
Johnston, B.F. 'Food, Health and Population in Deve-
    lopment', *Journal of Economic Literature*, vol.
    15, no.3 (1977), pp.879-907
Johnston, J. *Econometric Methods*, 2nd edn (McGraw
    Hill, New York, 1972)
Jones-Lee, M.W. *The Value of Life: An Economic Ana-
    lysis* (Martin Robertson, London, 1976)
Kallen, D.J. 'Nutrition and Society' (Paper Present-
    ed at the Conference on Nutrition and Human De-
    velopment, Michigan State University, East
    Lansing, 1969)
Kanawati, A.A. and D.S. McLaren, 'Failure to Thrive
    in Lebanon', *Acta Paediatrica Scandinavica*, vol.
    62,(1973), pp.571-576
Keeney, R. and H. Raiffa, *Decisions with Multiple
    Objectives: Preferences and Value Tradeoffs*
    (John Wiley, New York, 1976)
Kocher, J. and R.A. Cash, 'Achieving Health and Nu-
    tritional Objectives within a Basic Needs
    Framework' (Discussion Paper no.55, Harvard
    Institute for Economic Development, Boston,
    1979)
Koopman, J.S. 'Diarrhea and School Toilet Hygiene in
    Cali, Colombia', *American Journal of Epidemio-
    logy*, vol.107, no.5 (1978), pp.412-420
Kugelmass, N.L.,*et.al.* 'Nutritional Improvement of
    Child Mentality', *American Journal of the Medi-
    cal Sciences*, vol.218, (1944), pp.631-633
Kunstadter, P. 'Child Mortality and Maternal Parity:
    Some Policy Implications', *Int.Fam.Plann.Per-
    spect.Dig.*, vol.4, no.75 (1978)
Latham, L., M. Latham and S.S. Basta, 'The Nutritio-
    nal and Economic Implications of Ascaris Infec-

tion in Kenya' (World Bank Staff Paper no.271,
World Bank, Washington D.C., 1977)

Levine, R.J., *et.al.* 'Failure of Sanitary Wells to
Protect against Cholera and Other Diarrheas
in Bangladesh', *The Lancet*, vol.2, (1976), pp.
86-89

Levinson, F.J. 'Morinda: An Economic Analysis of
Malnutrition among Young Children in Rural
India' (International Nutrition Policy Series,
Cornell/MIT, Cambridge, Mass., 1974)

Mata, L. 'Breast-feeding: Main Promotor of Infant
Health', *The American Journal of Clinical Nutrition*, vol.31, (1978), pp.2058-2065

McEvers, N.C. 'Health and the Assault on Poverty in
Low Income Countries', *Social Science and Medecine*, vol. 14 C, (1980), pp.41-57

McLaren, D.S. and A.A. Kanawati, 'The Epidemiology
of Protein-Calorie Malnutrition in Jordan',
*Transactions of the Royal Society of Tropical
Medecine and Hygiene*, vol.64, no.5 (1970), pp.
754-768

Meegama, S.A. 'Malaria Eradication and Its Effect on
Mortality Levels', *Population Studies*, vol.21,
(1967), pp.207-237

——— 'The Decline in Maternal and Infant Mortality
and Its Relation to Malaria Eradication', *Population Studies*, vol.23, (1969), pp.289-302;
pp.305-306

Mooney, G.H., E.M. Russell and R.D. Weir, *Choices
for Health Care* (The MacMillan Press, London,
1980)

Morawetz, D. *Twenty-five Years of Economic Development* (The Johns Hopkins University Press, Baltimore, 1977)

Morley, D.C., *et.al.* 'Factors Influencing the Growth
and Nutritional Status of Infants and Young
Children in a Nigerian Village', *Transactions
of the Royal Society of Tropical Medecine and
Hygiene*, vol.62, no.2 (1968), pp.164-165

Morrow, R.H., *et.al.* 'A Quantitative Method of Assessing the Health Impact of Different Diseases
in Less Developed Countries', *International
Journal of Epidemiology*, vol.10, no.1 (1981),
pp.73-80

Mosley, W.H. 'Health, Nutrition and Mortality in
Bangladesh' in I. Sirageldin (ed.), *Research
in Human Capital and Development* (JAI Press,
Greenwich, Connecticut, 1979)

Mushkin, S.J. 'Health as an Investment', *Journal of
Political Economy*, vol.62 (Suppl.Oct.62), part

2, no.5 (1962)

Naylor, T.H. (ed.) *Computer Simulation Experiments with Models of Economic Systems* (John Wiley, New York, 1971)

Newman, P. 'Malaria Eradication and Population Growth with Special Reference to Ceylon and British Guyana' (Research Series no.10, Bureau of Public Health Economics, University of Michigan, School of Public Health, Ann Arbor, 1965)

—— 'Malaria Control and Population Growth', *Journal of Development Studies*, vol.6, no.2 (1970), pp. 138-158

—— 'Malaria and Mortality', *Journal of the American Statistical Association*, vol.72, no.358 (1977), pp.257-263

Omran, A.R. and C.C. Standley (eds.), *Family Formation Patterns and Health: An International Collaborative Study in India, Iran, Lebanon, Philippines and Turkey* (WHO, Geneva, 1976)

Orubuloye, I.O. and O.Y. Oyeneye, 'Primary Health Care in Developing Countries: The Case of Nigeria, Sri Lanka and Tanzania', *Social Science and Medecine*, vol.16, (1982), pp.675-686

Philippines Cholera Committee, *Field Evaluation of Environmental Sanitation Measures Against Cholera: Strategy and Cholera Control* (WHO, Geneva, 1971)

Prescott, N.M. 'The Economics of Malaria, Filariasis and Human Trypanosomiasis' (Working draft, Magdalen College, Oxford, 1979)

Puffer, R. and C.V. Serrano, 'Patterns of Mortality in Childhood' (Scientific Publication no.262, PAHO and WHO, Washington, 1973)

Rajesekaran, P., *et.al.* 'Impact of Water Supply on the Incidence of Diarrhea and Shigelloses among Children in Rural Communities in Madurai', *Indian Journal of Medical Research*, vol.66, no.2 (1977), pp.189-199

Rosenfield, P.L., R.A. Smith and M.G. Wolman, 'Development and Verification of a Schistosomiasis Transmission Model', *American Journal of Tropical Medecine and Hygiene*, vol.26, no.3 (1977), pp.505-516

Schliessman, D.J. 'Diarrheal Disease and the Environment', *Bulletin of the WHO*, vol.21, no.3 (1959), pp.381-386

Schneider, R.E., M. Schiffman and J. Faigenblum, 'The Potential Effect of Water on Gastrointestinal Infections Prevalent in Developing Countries', *The American Journal of Clinical Nutrition*, vol.

31, (1978), pp.2089-2099

Schultz, T.P. 'Interpretation of Relations among Mortality, Economics of the Household and Health Environment' (Meeting on Socio-Economic Determinants and Consequences of Mortality, Mexico City, 1979)

Scrimshaw, N.S. 'Malnutrition, Learning and Behavior', *American Journal of Clinical Nutrition*, vol.20, (1967), pp.493-502

Scrimshaw, N.S., *et.al.* *Interactions of Nutrition and Infection* (WHO, Geneva, 1968), pp.60-142

Seiler, K. *Introduction to Systems Cost-Effectiveness* (Wiley, New York, 1969)

Selowsky, M. and L. Taylor, 'The Economics of Malnourished Children: An Example of Disinvestment in Human Capital', *Economic Development and Cultural Change*, vol.22, no.1 (1973), pp.17-30

Sharpston, M.J. 'Health and Human Environment', *Finance and Development*, vol.13, no.1 (1976), pp.24-47

Sheehan, G. and M. Hopkins, *Basic Needs Performance: An Analysis of Some International Data* (ILO, Geneva, 1979)

Sommer, A. and M.S. Loewenstein, 'Nutritional Status and Mortality: A Prospective Validation of the QUAC Stick', *American Journal of Clinical Nutrition*, vol.28, (1975), pp.287-292

Sorkin, A.L. *Health Economics in Developing Countries* (Lexington Books, Lexington Mass.,1976)

Soysa, P.E. 'The Advantages of Breast-Feeding', *Assignment Children*, vol.55/56, (1981), pp.25-40

Spiegel, M.R. *Theory and Problems of Statistics* (McGraw Hill, New York, 1972)

Stanley, R. 'Water Supply Needs: An Integrated Approach', *The IDRC-Report*, vol.6, no.3 (1977), pp.11-14

Stephenson, L.S., M.C. Latham and M.L. Oduori, 'Costs, Prevalence and Approaches for Control of Ascaris Infection in Kenya', *Journal of Tropical Pediatrics*, vol.26, (December 1980), pp.246-263

Sterky, G., *et.al.* 'Challenges in Research on Tropical Diseases' (Swedish Agency for Research Co-operation with Developing Countries, Stockholm, 1977)

Stokey, E. and R. Zeckhauser, *A Primer for Policy Analysis* (Norton and Cy., New York, 1978)

Streeten, P.C.S. *First Things First - Meeting Basic Needs in Developing Countries* (Oxford University Press, Oxford, 1981)

Taylor, C.E. 'Stages in the Planning Process' in

W.E. Reinke (ed.), *Health Planning - Qualitative Aspects and Quantitative Techniques* (Waverley Press Inc., Baltimore, 1972)

Taylor, C.E.,*et.al. Malnutrition, Infection, Growth and Development: The Narangwal Experience* (World Bank and Johns Hopkins University Press, Baltimore, 1978)

Tripathy, K.,*et.al.* 'Effects of Ascaris Infection on Human Nutrition', *American Journal of Tropical Medecine and Hygiene*, vol.20, (1971), pp.212-218

—— 'Malabsorption Syndrome in Ascariasis', *American Journal of Clinical Nutrition*, vol.25, (1972), pp.1276-1281

Unido, *Guidelines for Project Evaluation* (United Nations, New York, 1972)

United Nations, *Yearbook of National Accounts Statistics 1979, vol.II* (United Nations, New York, 1980)

Van Gaelen, I. and W. Nonneman, 'Determinants of Health Status' (Working Paper no.7984, SESO, Antwerpen, 1979)

Van Zijl, W.J. 'Studies in Diarrheal Diseases in Seven Countries', *Bulletin of the WHO*, vol.35, no.2 (1966), pp.249-261

Vaughan, J.P. 'Are Doctors Always Necessary?', *Journal of Tropical Medecine and Hygiene*, vol. 21, (December 1971), pp.265-271

Wagner, E.G. and J.N. Lanoix, Excreta Disposal for Rural Areas and Small Communities' (WHO Monograph Series no.39, WHO, Geneva, 1958), p.22

Walsh, J.A. and K.S. Warren, 'Selective Primary Health Care: An Interim Strategy for Disease Control in Developing Countries', *The New England Journal of Medecine*, vol.301, no.18 (1979), pp.967-974

Wells, S. and W. Klees, *Health Economics and Development* (Praeger Studies, New York, 1980)

Wheeler, D. 'Basic Needs Fulfillment and Economic Growth: A Simultaneous Model', *Journal of Development Economics*, no.7 (1980), pp.435-451

Winikoff, B. and G. Brown, 'Nutrition, Population and Health: Theoretical and Practical Issues', *Social Science and Medecine*, vol.14 C (1980), pp.171-176

Winnick, M. and P. Rosso, 'The Effect of Severe Early Malnutrition on Cellullar Growth of Human Brain', *Pediatric Research*, no.3 (1969), pp.181-184

Wonnacott, R.J. and T.H. Wonnacott, *Introductory Statistics* (Wiley, New York, 1969)

—— *Econometrics* (Wiley, New York, 1970)
World Bank, *Atlas* (World Bank, Washington D.C.,
    1976a)
—— *Health Sector Policy Paper* (World Bank, Wash-
    ington D.C., 1980a)
—— *Village Water Supply* (World Bank, Washington
    D.C. 1976b)
—— *Atlas* (World Bank, Washington D.C., 1977)
—— *World Development Report 1978* (Oxford Univer-
    sity Press, Oxford, 1978)
—— *World Development Report 1979* (Oxford Univer-
    sity Press, Oxford, 1979)
—— *World Development Report 1980* (Oxford Univer-
    sity Press, Oxford, 1980b)
—— *World Development Report 1981* (Oxford Univer-
    sity Press, Oxford, 1981)
—— *World Development Report 1982* (Oxford Univer-
    sity Press, Oxford, 1982)
World Health Organization, 'Country Health Program-
    ming' (Report by the Director-General to the
    31st World Health Assembly, WHO, Geneva, 30
    March 1978)
Wray, J.D. and A. Aguirre, 'Protein-Calorie Mal-
    nutrition in Candelaria, Columbia', *Journal of
    Tropical Pediatrics*, vol.15, no.3 (1969), pp.
    79-88
Wray, J.D. 'Population Pressure on Families: Family
    Size and Child Spacing' in *Rapid Population
    Growth: Consequences and Implications* (Johns
    Hopkins University Press, Baltimore and London,
    1971), pp.462-478
—— 'Direct Nutrition Intervention and the Control
    of Diarrheal Disease in Malnourished Children'
    (Paper prepared for the National Academy of
    Sciences Workshop on Effective Interventions
    to Reduce Infections in Malnourished Populations,
    June 1977)
Wright, F.J. and J.P. Baird, *Tropical Diseases*,
    4th edn (Churchill Livingstone, Edinburgh and
    London, 1971)
Yayasuriya, D. and P.E. Soysa, 'Feeding Studies on
    Ceylonese Babies', *Journal of Environmental
    and Child Health*, vol.20, no.6 (1974), pp.275-
    279
Zeitlan, M.F. and C. Formacion, 'The HIID/UP-Col-
    lege Iloilo Evaluation of the Manoff Interna-
    tional Nutrition Education Radio Advertising
    Campaign in Iloilo, Philippines' (Harvard In-
    stitute for International Development, Boston,
    1978)

SUBJECT INDEX

add factor 151
attributes 102

base case simulation
    148
basic needs 6
basic needs model
    137-147
benefits and costs to
    society 53-55
birth spacing 11-12
body growth and mal-
    nutrition 14-15
bottom up planning
    process 171
breast feeding 8-9,14

calibration 150
coefficient of deter-
    mination 123
confidence interval 129
consumer's surplus 54
corner of the feasible
    region 115
cost-benefit analysis
    53-89
cost-effectiveness
    analysis 90-101
country health pro-
    gramming 162-171

days of healthy life
    lost 96-101
dependent variable 120
diseases 9-10

distribution weights 61,
    76
disturbance term 120,127
dominance 104-105
dummy variables 135

economic growth and
    health 3-5, 38-40
econometric modeling 136
education and nutrition
    17
estimator 123
equivalent alternatives
    105-108
expected net present
    value 62

feasible region 115
fertility 7,48

health development pro-
    grams 166
health planning 162-172
health strategy 165-166
housing and health 16
human capital 38

impact ratio 91
independent variable 120
indirect effects 62-63
infection and malnutri-
    tion 13
intangible benefits 58
intellectual development
    and malnutrition 15